THE WHITE COAT CHRONICLES

Anthology of Real Stories

Curated By

Sabeena Salam & Dr. Mariyam Thahira

notionpress.com

INDIA • SINGAPORE • MALAYSIA

ISBN
Paperback 979-8-90023-690-2
Hardcase 979-8-90136-636-3

CONTENTS

PART I: HEALING

**Tales from the hospital hallways,
engraved deep within healing hearts,
invoking courage, compassion, and comfort.**

PART II: LEARNING

Reflections on the journey of learning from thriving through medical schools to discovering unique paths.

A TRIBUTE

Striding into hospital corridors,
Your white coat worn as a badge of honour,
In your hands you hold a universe,
With a prayer to cure and create hope.

Amassing knowledge from both books and patients,
You seek to explore the world of medicine,
Your quiet struggles and daily sacrifices,
Some glimpsed by human eyes,
But all rewarded by our Creator.

May your smile and medical management,
Always stand shoulder to shoulder,
Let your words shine as glimmers of hope,
And may your compassion become a magical cure.

As we walk through the gardens of life,
Let us dream to change the world,
A kind word to our colleagues and,
A healing hand to our patients in need.

– Dr Faatimah Maryam Muzammil

PREFACE

Hospitals are often seen as places of diagnoses, prescriptions and procedures. But behind every white coat is a person, a human being navigating the fine line between strength and vulnerability. *The White Coat Chronicles* is a collection of stories that reveal the human side of medicine.

As someone who has always worked with words, I've long believed in the power of stories to heal, to connect, and to remind us of our shared humanity. Though I'm not a doctor myself, Narrative Medicine has always been close to me. Married to an ophthalmologist and sister to a nephrologist, I've heard countless stories over dinner tables, through late-night calls from hospitals, and quiet conversations when the weight of the day became too heavy to carry alone.

The inspiration for this collection was ignited during an engaging session I led with medical students at Dubai Medical University, where I introduced them to the transformative field of Narrative Medicine. While reflecting on powerful works that illuminate the emotional journeys of patients and the heart of healthcare, I also shared glimpses into my late brother's cherished library - a collection that quietly shaped him into a more compassionate physician and a profoundly thoughtful human being. As the session progressed, the students found echoes of their own experiences and of emotions felt but rarely named. In those stories, they recognised something vital: that writing could give voice to what medicine sometimes leaves unsaid.

Uncertain of the path but anchored by purpose, we began gathering narratives born from fleeting yet profound moments that reveal how, beneath every calm, clinical exterior, there beats a heart that feels deeply. These pages are not just reflections; they are reminders that healing is as much about humanity as it is about science.

Structured in two parts - *Healing and Learning* - the anthology captures both moments of compassion within hospital corridors and reflections on the process of medical education. The section on *Healing* highlights encounters that remind us of the power of empathy and compassion in the face of suffering. The section on *Learning* reflects on the journey of medical students and young doctors as they discover their calling, confront burnout, and navigate the complexities of professional identity.

Welcome to *The White Coat Chronicles*!

May these stories rekindle your faith in the practice of medicine, in the compassion we owe one another, and in the quiet, enduring truth that medicine, at its core, begins with humanity.

With hope and gratitude,

Mrs Sabeena Salam,

MPhil (English Literature & Applied Linguistics)

Educator | Advocate for compassionate learning

FOREWORD

It is with great honour and admiration that I write the foreword for the curated anthology *The White Coat Chronicles*. By bringing together diverse voices and stories, it has created a powerful testament to the human side of medicine.

As a Surgeon and Dean, I have had the privilege of witnessing the remarkable resilience of the human spirit. In my years of practice, I have come to understand that healing extends far beyond the physical restoration of the body. It encompasses the mind and spirit, woven together in the intricacies of human experience.

This anthology brings together voices from across the spectrum of medical practice: doctors, students, and trainees, each offering a glimpse into the lived realities of healthcare. Their narratives span moments of triumph and heartbreak, learning and unlearning, healing and loss. Together, these accounts form a mosaic of what it truly means to wear a white coat.

As you read these pages, you will be moved by the bravery of patients who confront their diagnoses with strength and grace. You will be inspired by the dedication of medical professionals who go above and beyond to provide comfort and care.

It is my hope that *The White Coat Chronicles* shall serve as a beacon of light for all who read it. For patients and their families, may these stories offer solace and strength. For healthcare professionals, may they serve as a reminder of the profound privilege and responsibility of our calling. And for all readers, may they foster a deeper appreciation for the resilience and integrity of the human spirit.

I extend my deepest gratitude to the contributors of this anthology for sharing their stories, and to the editors for bringing this remarkable collection to life. Together, you have created a work that will resonate deeply within the hearts of its readers and contribute to the ongoing dialogue about the power of Narrative Medicine. May these chronicles inspire and uplift you as much as they have done for me.

With heartfelt thanks and best wishes,

Dr Yousif Eltayeb, *MBBCh (Cairo), MSc (Sudan),*
FRCSI (Ireland), FRCS (UK), MIS (France),
Cert Med Edu (Keele, UK), Cert Leadership in Med Edu (HSD, USA)

Surgeon, Dean of the College of Medicine, Dubai Medical University.

DISCLAIMER

All names and identifying details of patients mentioned in this book have been changed to protect their privacy. The case descriptions are intended solely for educational and illustrative purposes, and care has been taken to ensure confidentiality in accordance with ethical standards.

No part of this book may be used as a substitute for professional medical advice.

CONTACT US

To share any feedback, suggestions, or ideas,
please reach out to
narratetoheal@gmail.com

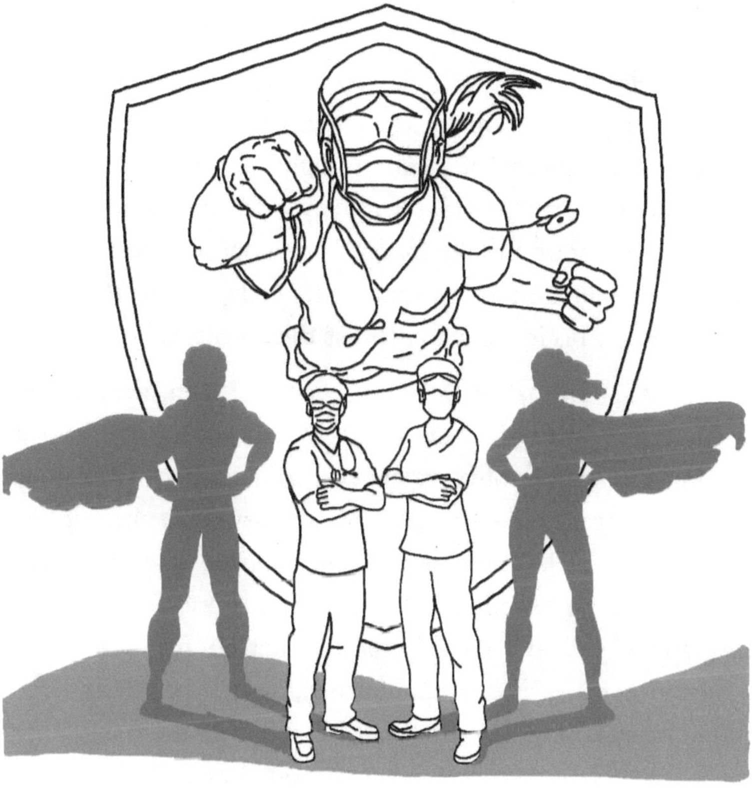

BRAVE
AND
BEYOND

A JOURNEY OF COURAGE

Dr Yousif Eltayeb

It was 1994 when I first met a particular patient who left an unforgettable mark on my heart. The diagnosis was breast cancer, a term that carries with it a heavy weight of fear and uncertainty. The news was delivered with the gravity it deserved. As I explained to her the diagnosis and the treatment options, her husband's face grew pale. Overcome by the shock, he collapsed on the floor, a stark reality of his inability to process the severity of the situation.

His wife (the patient), though visibly shaken, demonstrated a remarkable strength. She faced the diagnosis with a quiet determination, her resolve evident even as she began her treatment. Her journey was marked by an extraordinary resilience, especially as she faced not just one, but two *mastectomies*. The first surgery was a harrowing experience, both physically and emotionally, as she grappled with the loss of a part of herself. Just as she began to rebuild her life, the cancer returned, forcing her to undergo a second mastectomy. The prospect of enduring the trauma again was daunting, but she met it with remarkable strength. The second surgery, though equally challenging, became a turning point for her. Rather than succumbing to despair, she chose to channel her pain into a source of empowerment, both for herself and for others facing similar battles. Her experience of undergoing two mastectomies became a cornerstone of her advocacy, allowing her to connect deeply with other patients and to offer them hope and solace during their own journeys. Her journey through the challenges of cancer was marked not just by personal struggle but by a powerful will to overcome.

Even today, years later, she has transformed her own battle into a beacon of hope for others. By sharing her story, she became a source of solace for many patients grappling with similar fears. Her transition from patient to advocate was marked by her tireless efforts to connect with others going through the trauma of a cancer diagnosis.

She made it a mission to visit newly diagnosed patients, offering them a firsthand account of her own journey. Her presence was a calming force. She spoke with empathy and understanding, addressing their fears and uncertainties with a unique perspective born from her own experiences. Her ability to articulate the emotional and physical trials of cancer treatment provided a sense of companionship and hope.

One particular instance stands out. A young patient, newly diagnosed and overwhelmed by the prospect of treatment, connected with my initial patient. Through their conversation, she shared not only her own trials but also the triumphs she had experienced. She spoke of the long road to recovery, the moments of doubt, and her eventual victory over the disease. Her words were a balm to the young patient's anxious mind. Her influence extended even beyond one-on-one meetings. She organised support groups where patients could share their experiences and find strength in collective resilience. Her insights and encouragement fostered a community of support, where individuals could confront their fears in a nurturing environment. The groups she facilitated became a sanctuary for many, a place where they could find both practical advice and emotional support.

In reflecting on that patient's journey, I am continually inspired by how she has channelled her own experience into a force for good. Her transformation from a patient facing the unimaginable to a compassionate advocate has profoundly impacted the lives of those she has touched. Her legacy is one of courage and solace, offering a guiding light to others navigating their own paths through the tests of time. Her journey from a frightened patient to a compassionate supporter serves as a poignant reminder of the strength of the human spirit and the profound impact one person can have on the lives of many.

AGE IS JUST A NUMBER

Dr Sheeba Mariyam

Working as a general surgeon in a teaching hospital, I have attended to patients of various profiles across all age groups. The extremes of age have always been the most interesting. With children, the way they bounce back in the little while it takes medicine to act on their tiny bodies is nothing short of magical. Older patients, on the other hand, sometimes surprise you with unexpected outcomes. One such experience with a ninety-six-year-old lady was truly inspiring for me, both as a surgeon and as a person.

I've noticed that by age seventy, most people consider themselves old and start waiting to reach their eternal abode according to their beliefs. When older patients with emergent conditions and poor prognoses arrive, it is standard practice to discuss how far they are willing to go with medical and surgical interventions, unlike younger patients, for whom aggressive treatment is typically the default approach. The quality of life after intervention is what drives decisions in such cases.

When this ninety-six-year-old woman arrived, she had a history of colon cancer and had undergone surgery a decade earlier, resulting in an *end colostomy* (an opening for the colon through the abdomen). I am sure that the *oncology* surgeon must also have weighed these factors in mind while deciding to operate on an eighty-six-year-old back then.

Now, she was presenting with a perforated *parastomal hernia* (a hernia around the colostomy site) and impending shock, a situation that required urgent intervention. I discussed the available options with her and her children, despite my bias regarding age.

She said, "I've had a good run, even with the cancer. But I intend to continue fighting, so do what you can," to which her children gladly agreed. With an instant surge in respect for this lady, I prepared her for long hours of surgery where her aged heart and other organs gave my surgical team an adrenaline-fuelled experience. Despite all these factors, she continued to improve in the postoperative period. Her determination and strong-willed nature made me a stricter physician, making her work through her postoperative period as I would work with a younger patient. She surprised me at every step.

On her first postoperative outpatient visit, she came walking into the clinic, all cleaned up, immaculately dressed, and smelling of sandalwood. Seeing her, I was overjoyed. She had brought me some *unniyappam* (sweet rice cakes) that she had made herself. Although I have had many such experiences since, this one holds a special place in my heart.

RED-BUS STICKER

Dr Shaista Khadim

She clings to her little boy
As we tell her, "Your child has blood cancer."
She begins wailing
Then comes the sobbing
The silence ensues.

"Could we have prevented this?"
Asks the father with a shaking voice.
We shake our heads, and he looks away.

We break the silence
As we begin to talk about blood cancer
About the good prognosis it has
About all the other children we have treated in the past
About the management plan
And about how their child will make it through.

Her eyes explore our faces
Imploring us to tell her that this is all a misunderstanding
Her arms hold her boy tighter

His hands stroke his child's hair
His eyes glistening with tears that can't make their way out
And their hands holding each other tightly as we talk.

I look at the little boy
Sitting calmly in his mother's lap
Exploring the red-bus sticker we gave him
Unaware of how the world has come crashing down for his parents,
Innocently enjoying the tight hug his mother gives him.

And I wonder:
Maybe this is what will help the parents pull through
The dream of what their child can be in the future
The faith that their child will make it through
The hope that not all is lost

Painfully and slowly, they calm down
Shoulders relaxing
Eyes bloodshot but not teary anymore
The hug and handholding loosen a little
As we near the end of the conversation, they smile,
"He will make it through"

And we nod. We smile.
He will make it through.

LANDING ON THE MOON

Dr Srutdi Kamalam Natarajan

I had a professor who always told us that our patients are our best teachers. I always assumed it meant gaining knowledge in a clinical setting. Maybe it does, because reality is harsh and an excellent teacher. But there is more to that statement.

I still remember my very first conversation with a patient who taught me lessons far more valuable than medicine. She had been admitted with *Beta-Thalassemia*, a type of *anaemia* requiring lifelong transfusions. When I entered her room to take history, she sat up, eyes bright and proclaimed, "Hi, Doctor! I have Beta-Thalassemia!" I was very confused and amused at the same time. Yet, I proceeded to smile, asked her a few questions about how she was feeling, and collected her history. She has been receiving blood transfusions for almost fifteen years now. Every time I looked at her, I saw her hopeful eyes and joyful smile, which never dissipated. Her positive attitude brought me a great deal of comfort and joy, and we became acquainted in no time.

One day, I asked her, "So, tell me, what do you want to become when you grow up?"

"A lawyer? Maybe a teacher? Or I might even start a business," she said eagerly. I laughed at her enthusiastic response. "You know what they say, aim for the moon, even if you miss, you'll land among the stars," I responded encouragingly. Her face turned defiant. "Doctor, I will land on the moon," she replied, with quiet determination.

Well, that was new - something I never thought of myself. I took a moment to introspect on what she had said. What exactly is the moon? Why were we told to aim for the moon and settle for something that's not the moon? Why did I believe the moon is unattainable? Of course, the stars might be beautiful and worthy, too, but I know that I am invariably setting my goal to be out of reach, and I just hope to settle for something close enough. The moon doesn't have to be anything extraordinary. It is simply something that you truly desire. It is what you're willing to work for and the purpose you want to fulfil. The moon is exactly where you want to be.

"Aim for the moon and make sure you land on it," I told her as I handed her the discharge papers.

THE BEAUTY OF A NEW LIFE

Dr Shabana Muzammil

It was during my *internship* year that I truly embodied the spirit of becoming a doctor. Rotating in different departments helped me develop insight into unique cases and challenging patients. As I was rotating through my *Obstetrics and Gynaecology (OBGYN)* rotation, I came across a homeless lady who was pregnant and severely malnourished. She was admitted to our hospital, and one morning, while doing rounds, she suddenly went into *labour*. She delivered the baby and started bleeding profusely. Our entire team of doctors attended to her critical condition, but she went into *shock* and passed away.

The new challenge our team now faced was the little being before us. She kept crying, and our dedicated team of nurses tried various things to calm her down. Hearing this tiny life cry in desperation changed something in me that day. I gathered the courage and spoke to the Head of the Department, requesting permission to take care of this baby's needs. He smiled and agreed but placed a condition, stating that the baby could not be taken out of the hospital at any cost, to which I agreed. I started a small initiative of collecting funds from my college friends and other doctors in the hospital to take care of this child.

As time passed, the baby was growing, and so were her needs. I named her "Pari," which means Angel. Pari became a part of our morning rounds, and the entire team would make sure to smile and play with her for a few minutes. I still remember that she was adorable and cheerful all the time. I felt a deep sense of responsibility towards her and realised that my internship in this hospital would soon come to an end. I wanted to take steps to ensure a secure future for her. As her identity could not be traced back, I realised she needed a forever home. I was truly grateful that the hospital management had allowed us to take care of her for an extended period of time, but also knew this period would not last forever. So, I decided to visit an orphanage centre to register her for adoption.

As time went by, Pari continued to grow, and so did the fear in my heart. Her adoption process did not seem to work out. I kept praying for her, and one fine day, it felt like the Creator did a miracle. I found a couple who were willing to adopt Pari after four and a half months of desperate searching. She was finally adopted legally. The day she finally left our ward was filled with joy and pain. We were overjoyed that she found a forever home, yet saddened by her departure. Now, my Head of the Department placed a condition on me that henceforth he would keep in touch with the parents, and I should not disturb them. With a little bit of resistance, I agreed. He wanted me as a student to focus on my career and life.

Pari's story remains with me to this day. She was my first real lesson in the responsibility that comes with this profession, and since then, I have promised myself to always approach my patients with the same dedication and heart that she first inspired in me. This incident impacted me to the level that I went on to practice in the OBGYN field for around a decade. It was truly momentous for me to see children being born and bringing smiles to the faces of their families.

Life gives us so many opportunities to learn and create an impact in one's life. As a doctor, I saw many things happen and change. I truly believe that the essence of our responsibility towards our patients should always remain the same. We should never let go of our oath to practice medicine to serve people. I believe that life is a precious gift of the Almighty. We should work towards saving and improving it endlessly for the benefit of humanity. My advice to all doctors practising medicine is to love what you do and do what you love.

WHO IS A DOCTOR?

Dr Abrar Dhaifallah Alameri

Tuesday morning, 9:35 a.m. – just a regular day in the *dermatology* clinic, buzzing with the chaos of back-to-back appointments of patients following up for their acne treatment on a busy day. Today is going to be an acne-only day, or so I thought.

Amidst the shuffle of patients, a man entered our clinic, barely walking, without carrying a cane or crutches, using his hands and sidebars to aid his injured foot in walking. His discomfort became evident with every slow step. As a medical student, I've been taught to notice the small things, to observe how a patient enters the room. His gait was laboured, his body heavy with the weight of his struggles, both physical and emotional. He clutched a grocery bag, filled not with food but with his entire identity: medical reports, personal documents, as if he were carrying the burdens of his life in that single plastic bag. I approached to help him onto a seat. He let out a sigh of frustration, one that had probably been building up for months, maybe years.

His complaint was simple: a *nodule* on the sole of his left foot. But nothing is ever that simple in medicine. He came because that small lump was the latest roadblock in a life full of obstacles. Recently diagnosed with *diabetes*, he was desperate to avoid medication, determined to lose weight and reclaim his health. But this tiny, stubborn nodule was preventing him from carrying out even the slightest form of physical activity.

After a thorough history and examination, the doctor suggested a *biopsy*. He refused; his words were sharp and desperate. We tried to reassure him, promising that the procedure would be quick and almost painless, but his refusal grew louder, more urgent. Grabbing his bag, he prepared to leave.

As he left the room, the doctor quietly followed. A few minutes later, the office phone rang. I answered, and on the other end, a nurse from the procedure room asked, "Did the patient for the foot biopsy pay the fee?"

Suddenly, everything clicked into place.

I overheard another nurse reply, "The doctor said she'll take care of it."

"She'll probably pay for it herself," the first nurse replied.

"Okay, thank you, dear. Bye."

At that moment, I felt something shift inside me. You would think*: Oh, what a lucky patient, it's his lucky day to come to this doctor.* However, my initial reaction was: *Wow! What a lucky doctor!*

You might be wondering what I mean by lucky doctor? Lucky to have the means and the heart to act. Not that the doctor's duty itself isn't enough of giving a hand in changing patients' lives, but to be someone who does it from their heart, for their patients, not just because it is their job. And the fact that the nurses were not surprised meant that she had done this before for other patients. It was then that I understood the true weight of what it means to be a doctor.

It's not just about treating a disease; it's about treating the person as a whole, which can affect the whole community. The small things, the quiet refusal of care, speak volumes about a patient's life. As in this case, sometimes, the most important medicine we can offer is our willingness to help, without hesitation or judgement.

"SUPER SURGEONS: A CHANCE AT LIFE" – A PERSONAL REFLECTION

Dr Vinidh Paleri

When the team from Wonderhood Studios approached me about filming "Super Surgeons: A Chance at Life," a documentary series for Channel Four in partnership with The Royal Marsden, I wasn't sure what to say.

Surgeons aren't used to the spotlight. We work quietly, often anonymously, behind sterile drapes and closed theatre doors. Our focus is the patient - always the patient - not the camera. Every decision on the table, every cut with the *scalpel* or *cautery* blade is carefully planned, with the mind contemplating the next steps of the procedure. Allowing cameras into the theatre environment, to witness and record that process, felt vulnerable.

But then I thought of the people who come through our doors, people who are facing unthinkable diagnoses with quiet determination. People who say yes to life when everything seems to say no. If this series could even begin to tell their stories - honestly, respectfully - then maybe it was worth accepting that as a trade-off.

What followed was one of the most humbling experiences of my career. Super Surgeons doesn't dramatise what we do. It doesn't create miracles. Instead, it captures the raw, often unspoken truth of complex cancer care - the sweat, the intricate planning before complex operations, the unexpected setbacks and the need to think on our feet, the long silences, and the hard-won victories. It shows the precision of surgery to give someone a second chance at life.

One patient's story still stays with me. The diagnosis was aggressive, the surgery invasive, the reconstruction daunting. It was the kind of case that tests not just your training, but your humanity. But what I remember most is the patient's spirit - unwavering even in the face of pain. That kind of bravery humbles you. The cameras captured it, but the memory lives deeper than any frame of film.

I'm grateful I was a part of it. Because this series isn't about surgeons, it's about people. About resilience. About what it means to be broken and to heal. About the sacred space between fear and hope, and those who stand in that space, trying their best to help.

If "Super Surgeons" helps even one person walk into a consultation a little less afraid or helps one loved one understand the battle a bit more clearly, then those open theatre doors were worth it!

GOING THE EXTRA MILE

Dr Afrah Ghayoor

It was yet another busy day in the *Gynaecology* ward, with constant calls and tasks pulling me from all directions. Amidst all the chaos, though, one patient stood out, her case silently tugging at my heartstrings.

A young housemaid had presented with severe pain in the lower abdomen and fever. Upon further investigation, she was diagnosed with *Pelvic Inflammatory Disease (PID)* complicated by an ovarian *abscess.* Although her infection was severe, her only concern was about leaving the hospital, as she couldn't afford the treatment.

Seeing her in that distraught state bothered me. Yet, overwhelmed by the flurry of tasks that lay ahead of me, my unease got buried beneath the caverns of yet another exhausting day. A part of me was resigned, ready to fill the form of *'Discharge Against Medical Advice' (DAMA)*, which she could sign before insistently leaving. Another part of me, though, just felt helpless; I was new to the hospital and unaware of its policies and possibilities in providing care amidst financial and social barriers.

A little later, the same day, I was pulled from my work by a call from one of the nurses covering the same ward that day. She was concerned that the patient's condition had worsened and urged me to reassess her. As our previous interactions had bred some mistrust, I was about to dismiss her point. Yet, something in her voice made me pause. She genuinely believed that the patient was sicker than we had initially thought. Thus, trusting my intuition, I rushed to check on the patient.

Upon reassessing her, I was faced with a distressing dilemma. On one hand, it was clear that the patient's condition had worsened, making it unsafe for her to leave and seek treatment elsewhere. On the other hand, her sponsor refused to pay for the treatment, and she simply couldn't afford it on her own. Anxious and desperate, she began insisting on being discharged on oral medications instead. However, understanding her condition, we knew they wouldn't be enough to manage the severity of the infection she was battling.

Caught between wanting to treat the patient and struggling to facilitate her hospital stay, I felt overcome by a mixture of guilt, confusion, and frustration. Feeling challenged, I began racking my brain for any possible solution.

It occurred to me then that the hospital might have social services or connections with charitable organisations that could help cover the cost of her treatment. Upon discussing the possibility with the nurse, I was overjoyed to find out that we could, in fact, request financial assistance.

Much to our relief, the social support team was willing to accept the patient and help cover the cost! We couldn't wait to reveal the news to her.

Once we conveyed it, the patient's reaction was unforgettable, her relief tangible. She felt as if we had untangled all her fears and unravelled the tight knot of despair that had taken hold of her.

Touched by our efforts and care, her eyes softened and filled with tears. "This feels like a miracle," she whispered, having already abandoned any hope of healing and recovery. Moved by her heartfelt expression, I found myself pausing to reflect on both the day's events and my approach towards it all.

This could have easily been another case dismissed as *'DAMA'* with a quick signature - another task cleared from a list where a whole host of other patients awaited care. Rushing from patient to patient, sometimes, it is quite easy to become desensitised, especially towards those who come with complexities that place us in dilemmas such as these.

While the initial inclination may be to dismiss and justify it with the weight of the demands upon us, sometimes, taking a moment to connect and empathise with our patients can transform the kind of care we are able to provide. Often, we're able to play a part in 'miracles' like these - not because of superpowers, vast knowledge, or impeccable skill, but simply because we care deeply about our patients' physical pain and emotional distress. That genuine concern is what pushes us to go the extra mile. And who knows - perhaps a leap of faith fuelled by empathy is all it takes to make a real difference in someone's life.

PSYCHED OUT!

Dr Riya Azeez and Dr Faatimah Maryam Muzammil

It was one of those days when I reported a bit later than I was supposed to. I was the on-call intern posted in *Psychiatry* for the day. As I reached the department, I noticed that the security guard positioned outside was not there. I reached out for the latch to open the main cell, which leads to the ward. Instantly, my eyes met a large, burly patient struggling to get away from two staff nurses, two nursing assistants, and an allied health student. They were trying to prevent him from reaching the main cell, but they were no match for the six-foot, heavy-set man who was now advancing towards me.

"Close the main cell," one of the nurses shouted out to me.

With trembling fingers, I pulled back the latch with all my might. I froze in fear as he glared at me. He reached out for the latch and began to open it. The blood drained from my face, and my hands and feet felt ice-cold. How I wished this was all just a bad dream. The click of the latch resonated in my ears, and reality forced me back into my senses. Gathering the last bit of courage, I turned around and bolted to the clinic next door, realising that I had to inform the receptionist.

I burst into her room and frantically repeated these lines, "Chechi, (word for sister in Malayalam), call the security immediately, a patient is about to abscond."

I had just completed the sentence when I felt someone whizz past me. The patient had absconded already! The receptionist yanked the telephone. "CODE BROWN, CODE BROWN," she yelled into the receiver. Code brown is activated when an adult patient goes missing from the hospital premises. A few seconds passed as we watched an allied health student chase after him. Without a second thought, I took off right behind him, following the patient down the stairs, out of the ward, and into the ground-floor medicine block. By now, our trio had caught the attention of the bystanders. Some of them even volunteered to run along to catch the patient, but he had almost reached the exit.

The allied health student called out to the guard, "Close the exit."

Unfortunately, it was too late. Despite the guards' attempts to shut the door, the patient overpowered them and forced open the doors. He then ran out of the building and towards the emergency medicine block. By then, Code brown had already taken effect. The security guards at all exit points were alerted, and the message had been wired to the entire hospital staff to look out for a 'male patient wearing a green T-shirt and shorts who is headed towards the emergency medicine block.'

The group of people chasing the man continued to expand. Amidst the chaos and commotion, however, we could hear the sound of the train at a distance; it was about to reach the railway crossing next to the hospital.

A chilling thought crossed my mind immediately, "Where was the patient headed?" There were a number of alarming possibilities that made me recognise the gravity of the situation. Left unguarded, a patient of this nature could easily fall into different kinds of harm outside, reminding me of our responsibility in protecting our patients. I just hoped ardently that he would be brought to a halt soon.

As a safety measure, five security guards were positioned at the emergency medicine block, but to their surprise, the patient swiftly took a left turn towards the auto rickshaw stand, skilfully dodging the guards. Minutes later, he was caught off guard by an oncoming scooter rider, which finally slowed him down. This gave the guards the right opportunity to stop him. A crowd had gathered around them, with everyone talking amongst each other about the mysterious man. Assumptions and theories filled the air.

I overheard one of them say, "Is it a thief?"

"Not sure," replied the other.

The speculations were quickly dismissed, and the patient was safely escorted into a car and taken back to the block. I heaved a sigh of relief as I saw the car pull into the block, realising that the patient was taken back to the *Psychiatry* department. He was then taken to his room and comforted by his bystander. Everyone looked at each other in the ward as silence overtook the department. Yet, deep down, we were just grateful that we could bring the patient back to the department safely. Worn out from the morning ordeal, I sank into the chair next to the main cell and pondered over the day's activities.

This internship has truly enabled me to experience many events that helped enhance my view of life. It has enjoined values like empathy and compassion for our patients, as well as the importance of responding quickly to unforeseen challenges. As much as this year has been academically enriching, the values and morals I have learned while training in this profession have also helped me grow and develop as a human being.

I gently closed my eyes and smiled to myself, while wondering what adventures would be in store for me tomorrow.

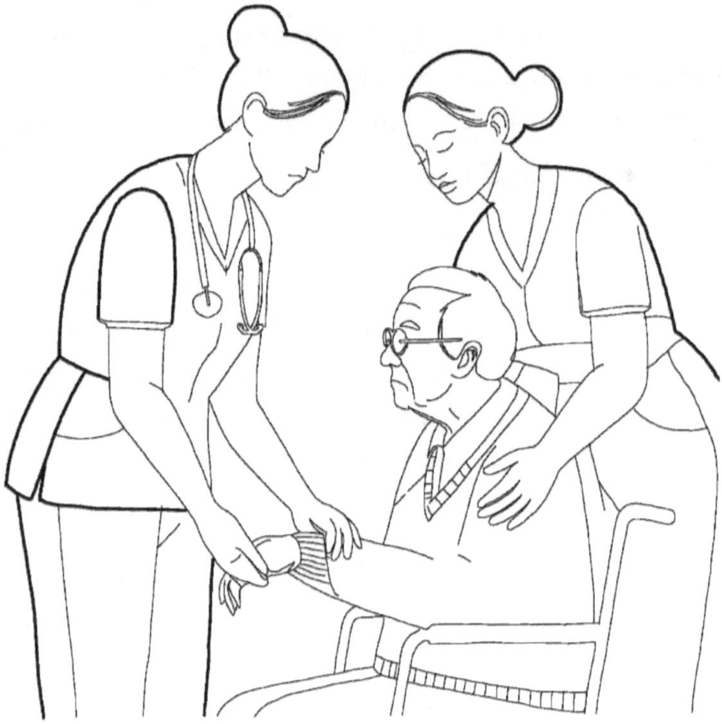

TRUST, TRANSFORMATION AND TOUCH

A CHILD'S SILENT STRUGGLE

Dr Suhaila Ahmed

"This child presented to the emergency department with sudden weakness in all four limbs," the doctor announced during our morning rounds. Half asleep, these words jolted me awake, igniting a mix of anticipation and curiosity within me. *Paediatrics* has always been fascinating to me, and through my clinical years, I have seen dozens of interesting cases, but nothing could have prepared me for the raw reality I was about to witness that day.

As I stepped into the hospital room, I was immediately struck by the scene before me. A little girl, not more than five years of age, lay still on the bed, her body almost ghostly in its silence. Her face was ashen, her mouth gaping, and her eyelids droopy. Her mother stood beside her, radiating an unexpected calm amidst the chaos. It was then that I knew that this was not the first time this child had gone limp. The mother's eyes were filled with a mix of worry and concern, while the child's eyes held a haunting emptiness that spoke volumes of her silent struggle. I could see the dried tears on her cheeks, a testament to her battle.

The mother began to recount the history of her daughter's condition. She explained that her child had been diagnosed with a rare disorder that caused her limbs to go limp without warning. She would be playing happily, then suddenly go limp in half of her body. These episodes had occurred intermittently over the years, leading to a life filled with uncertainty. However, this particular episode was different; for the first time, all four of her limbs had failed her. The child's mother spoke with a sense of both frustration and resilience, describing the many times they had been rushed to the hospital, seeking answers and relief.

As I examined the girl, a wave of empathy washed over me. Her face, once filled with the innocence and joy of childhood, was now a mask of emotions she could not express. I gently reached out to hold her hand, but her fingers were limp and unresponsive. I wrapped my hand around her tiny fingers, hoping to bridge the gap between us, even if it was just for a moment.

At that moment, the reality of her situation struck me profoundly. Here was a child who could see the world around her but couldn't engage with it. She could feel sadness but couldn't cry; she was trapped in a body that felt like it had betrayed her. It was heartbreaking. I could only imagine the fear that gripped her. I glanced over at her parents, whose desperation was palpable, yearning to understand and comfort their daughter while navigating the uncertainty of her condition.

Leaving the room, I couldn't shake the lingering sadness that enveloped me. My mind raced with thoughts about what I had just witnessed. How could a child, so full of potential, be reduced to this state? I quickly reviewed her medical notes with my resident, eager to learn more about the condition that had brought this family to the brink of despair. The diagnosis was *Alternating Hemiplegia of Childhood*, a rare neurological condition characterised by episodes of paralysis and developmental challenges. My heart sank further as I learned there was no known cure yet.

The next day, I returned to the hospital, unsure of what I would find. Walking down the familiar corridor, I felt a mix of apprehension and hope. Would I see the same girl who had been so motionless the day before? To my surprise, the little girl was no longer lying still. Instead, she was sitting up in bed, smiling brightly, her feet dancing with newfound energy. It was a remarkable transformation. Her mother beamed with relief, sharing tales of incremental progress. "She's been doing better today," her mother explained, her voice filled with a mix of joy and disbelief.

This shift in her condition was heartening and served as a powerful reminder of the resilience that childhood embodies. As I approached her bed, the girl's eyes sparkled with excitement. She remembered me as the doctor who held her hand the day before, and as I offered her some colourful stickers, her face lit up with joy. The stickers were a small gesture, but they seemed to brighten her spirits, allowing a glimpse of the child I had hoped to see.

However, just as I was about to leave, I noticed a change in her expression. Tears welled up in her eyes, and she reached out to me, silently pleading for me to stay. My heart swelled at the sight of her vulnerability. I knelt beside her, soothing her with soft words and gentle touches. "I'm right here. Don't worry," I assured her, hoping to calm her racing heart. It was a moment where the impact of a simple gesture - holding her hand - unveiled the profound power of human connection.

I couldn't help but reflect on how crucial the human touch is in our lives. In a world increasingly dominated by technology and automation, there was something irreplaceable about the warmth of a hand in another's. As a medical intern, I often found myself buried in textbooks, studying complex conditions and treatments. But here, in this small hospital room, I was reminded that sometimes healing goes beyond medicine; it resides in the bonds we form with others.

I watched the girl as she played with the stickers, her laughter filling the room. I felt a wave of gratitude wash over me, knowing I had been part of a moment that brought her joy amidst her struggles. Her spirit was infectious, and I realised how important it is to cherish these moments, not just in the hospital, but in life itself.

As I left the room, I carried with me a profound lesson. The small act of holding a child's hand made a difference not only in her day but in my heart as well. It was a reminder of the importance of compassion and connection, a fleeting glimpse of hope in the midst of hardship.

SOMETIMES, IT'S ALL ABOUT THE PRESENCE

Dr Fathima Aaliya Anwar

During my *internship* in the *OBGYN* department, an evening round was interrupted by an urgent call from the emergency room. A south-Asian patient at thirty-four weeks of pregnancy was in *septic abortion*, and I accompanied my doctor to assess the situation. In the *emergency room (ER)*, we saw a frail, semi-conscious, exhausted young woman being prepared for admission to the operating theatre. Meanwhile, her visibly anxious husband paced back and forth nervously.

Amid the chaos, I noticed a nurse struggling to obtain consent for the emergency procedure she had to undergo due to a language barrier. Seeing his confusion, I offered to step in. Speaking to him in his language, I explained the procedure, its purpose, and the associated risks. Gradually, his demeanour shifted from panic to a semblance of calm as he processed the information.

While I was walking towards the operating theatre, he stopped me.

"Could I stay with my wife during the procedure?"

I gently explained that hospital policy didn't allow it. What he said next left a lasting impression on me. He asked if I was performing the procedure, and I clarified that as an intern, I wasn't permitted to do so but reassured him that his wife was in expert hands.

What moved me deeply was his heartfelt request: even though I wasn't the one performing the procedure, he wanted me to be present in the operating room. He believed that my presence would offer his wife a sense of care, that she wouldn't just feel like another case file.

That moment was a profound reminder of the power of human connection. Sometimes, the greatest comfort we can provide isn't through our medical knowledge or skills, but through the simple act of being there. Reassurance and empathy can heal in ways that medicine alone cannot.

A JOURNEY IN DISCOVERY

Dr Maya Elmaghraby

On my first day of medical school, I remember the crack of dawn outside the imposing doors of the hospital, looking and feeling great in that crisp new white coat. My heart was pounding to the rhythm of excitement and trepidation because this was it, and today was the day - the beginning of a journey - a journey that could change my life in ways I could hardly have imagined.

The orientation ceremony was a blur of welcome words and inspiring speeches, but one line from the dean stuck with me: "You are about to embark on a voyage which will challenge you, break you, and rebuild you. Medicine is not just a profession; it is a calling, a commitment to the well-being of others." I didn't know then how prophetic his words would be.

The first year flew by in a flurry of lectures, labs, and late-night study sessions. *Anatomy* was particularly gruelling. The body in front of me in the dissection lab hit my senses like a jolt, a harsh reminder of the critical nature of the field I had chosen. The first incision had me shaking all over, but soon enough, I was comforted by the realisation that every cut I made led me closer to a deeper understanding of the human body.

Clinical rotations were a different beast. The transition from books to real patients was just daunting. I remember the first rotation in the *emergency* department: baptism by fire. The chaos, the urgency, and the sheer number of sufferers; there was nothing it could compare to. It was during this time that I experienced my first patient loss: a young man, not much older than myself, who died due to severe trauma. His face haunted me in my sleep for weeks after, a constant reminder of how fragile life truly was.

One experience that I recall during my volunteer work at a local clinic in my home country was when I was approached to assist a single mother, Maryam, who could not afford the healthcare for her children. All her efforts were focused on securing basic necessities for her children. Her strength and determination left an indelible mark on me. With the help of the clinic's assistance programmes, I got the chance to witness firsthand how access to quality healthcare truly transformed Maryam and her family's lives.

At the time, I was amazed by just how dramatically healthcare professionals could influence the lives of individuals as well as entire communities. Undoubtedly, among so many difficult moments, there were lots of truly eye-opening ones.

Definitely, one of my most memorable experiences was shadowing a *Paediatric oncologist.* During this time, I had the brief opportunity to meet a youngster whose courage and will to survive against all odds left a deep impression on me. The high level of his bright spirit and his never-to-die attitude, his unwavering determination to fight his illness, inspired one and all around him. Being surrounded by such tender care from the medical team within an environment created to be encouraging, he was as positive as could be, facing his treatment with courage and optimism. His experience only reaffirmed my desire to work in a field where I could make a difference in people's lives, just as these medical professionals had done for him.

Furthermore, my mentor has played a crucial role in my development. He is a brilliant surgeon with a heart of gold, blending professional skill and compassion seamlessly. He would always say to me, "Medicine is an art as much as a science. Never forget to treat the person, not merely the disease." With that advice,

I learned not only the details of surgery, but also how to present myself, to listen to patients, and to win their trust.

After another endless day in the operating theatre, my mentor invited me for an evening cup of coffee and said to me, "Every patient you treat is somebody's loved one. Remember that. Our call extends from the inside of the operating theatre. It's about making a difference in their life, no matter how small."

The second year of medical school brought a new set of challenges and learning opportunities. *Pharmacology* became very detailed, with the complexity of understanding the interaction of chemicals and the mechanism of their activity requiring a different type of intellectual exertion. Much of my time in medical school was spent reading textbooks and trying to memorise countless lists of drugs and their side effects. Somewhere in this period, I began to appreciate the level of precision and attention to detail required in medicine.

Amongst those rotations, the one that was most profound for me was *Psychiatry*. It was the intricacies and vulnerabilities of the human mind that really pulled me in. I remember working with a patient who had been fighting severe depression for years. It was through our sessions that I began to realise the depth of impact that mental illness can bring upon someone's life and the empathetic patience required to counter it. It was a slow and stumbling road to recovery for him, but with compassionate care, every small triumph proved his inner strength.

Another significant experience stemmed from my time in the surgical ward. The high-powered environment was both invigorating and intimidating. I assisted in quite a wide array of procedures, ranging from simple *appendectomies* to complex *vascular surgery* cases. The need for specificity and coordination in surgery is indicative of the importance of teamwork when working in any situation. Every successfully conducted surgery was huge, underlining advancements in medical science and the vitality and potential of skilled surgeons.

During my *Internal Medicine* rotation, I met a patient who changed my outlook towards patient care – an elderly lady suffering from several *chronic* conditions that made her a frequent visitor to the hospital. Given her weak condition, she was warm, gentle, and full of good words to share with whoever came near her. I spent many hours at her bedside, listening to her stories and learning about her life. Despite all her health issues, she remained so resilient and cheerful. She helped me understand that being a good doctor is not just about the treatment of diseases but about touching the human aspect in every patient, being able to understand the fears and hopes of each and providing them comfort and support.

My Paediatric rotation was a true rollercoaster ride, involving both joyful and heartbreaking moments. Children, filled with energy and innocence, showcased a totally different aspect of patient care. I would never forget the day I met a girl who was five years old and very ill with a complicated *congenital* heart disease. Despite her condition, she was an interactive and vivacious life force, always laughing and smiling. Her parents, worried down to the soul, were her unfaltering pillars of belief. It was through working with her that the importance of hope and the profound role of family support in healing were really highlighted.

As time went by in medical school, the importance of working in interprofessional teams was something that became strikingly obvious. I worked with a very well-rounded team of health professionals: nurses, pharmacists, social workers, and physical therapists. Each of these members brought a different perspective and expertise that aided our provision of holistic care to our patients. This not only boosted our patients' recovery but also enriched my understanding of holistic care.

Reflecting back on my journey, I think of the many mentors and role models that have shaped my serpentine path towards wisdom. Their experience, guidance and dedication to patient care have been instilled in my mind. They taught me that medicine is a lifelong pursuit of becoming better and aiming higher. Their love for medicine and the compassion they showed to patients invoked in me the desire to be the best doctor I could be.

As I stand here today, a fully-fledged physician, I glance back at the journey, both contented and grateful. No longer am I clothed in this white coat in its pure form; Every stain and wrinkle has a tale of its own - one of struggle, education, and compassion.

Studying medicine provided me with priceless insights into human nature, resilience, and the deep interconnection of human lives. I have seen the best and worst of human nature, but through it all, I learned empathy, humility, and the value of continuous learning. "White Coat Chronicles" is more than an anthology; it is a prism through which our collective experiences can be reflected on, and our journeys in pursuit of healing recognised.

My story is a small strand of this intricate tapestry and, hopefully, will inspire others as much as it has enriched my life. The career of a medical professional is endless. There are new challenges accompanying every new day, bringing chances for growth and maturity. As I continue winding my way through the twisted alleys of the medical world, I bear with me the lessons and memories of those who have touched my life. Their stories are woven into the fabric of me, guiding me as I endeavour to make a difference, one patient at a time.

With "The White Coat Chronicles," the hope is to do justice to those who came before me and give meaning to those just starting their own adventures within the world of medicine. This is mine, my chronicle, and it is only the beginning.

BURNING LIFE INTO COLOURS

Dr Anaam Parveen

No one warned us what the clinical side of medical school really meant. They spoke of it as the 'fun part,' a promised thrill after the grind of books and sleepless nights. The hospital where we began our very first clinical rotation felt nothing like a hospital. It felt more like stepping into a bustling mall, filled with splashes of colour and warmth that chased away any gloom, even if it was breeding deep within.

At the end of that first day, it wasn't a wind or a hailstorm even; it was a single huge cube of ice that we slammed face-first into reality - a single nose-breaking blow that shattered the illusion. My partner and I walked into the colourful wards with nerves and hopes swirling together like butterflies, only to watch them drop dead by the day's end, replaced by a bitter, gritty truth. In a team of *attendings, residents*, and interns, we weren't butterflies that people turned heads to here - just houseflies, hovering unnoticed, clinging to scraps of experience in a world too vast and busy to notice the two buzzing medical students.

I love to talk - a constant buzz of thoughts and questions - but my fellow medical student, not so much. Yet somehow, the silence of those long, sterile hours where we gowned, gloved, walked in and out of rooms and sanitised on repeat had even her itching to speak. By the time we escaped for a break, it was like our mouths were starved, words spilling out like a dam had burst, filling the air with everything we hadn't said in the last five hours. Every patient we saw, every observation we made, little details to the parts of stories we heard and kept patching together. We were like broken radios finally catching a signal, voices overlapping, desperately filling the empty space, clawing our way out of the stillness to the surface just to breathe.

The reality hit harder with each passing day, like a shadow that just grows longer as the sun dips at the horizon. At first, we brushed it off - maybe it was just a bad day, then two bad days. Surely, things would ease up. And when that hope frayed, we did what was left - trust in a plan we couldn't see, holding onto it as the days stacked up and the weight refused to lift. It pressed down when a week went by, and we finally grasped it: this was "the breeze" part of medical school everyone had raved about, the so-called easy stage. But there was nothing breezy about it. Coming to terms with that felt like seeing our cotton candy dissolve in the pond, replaced by air that left us empty.

From then on, everything grew quieter, like a song slipping into silence, leaving only the faintest hum behind. Gone were the butterflies, the flickers of anticipation. We moved through each day as ghosts, unseen and unheard, floating just beyond the edges of attention. There was no space for our voices here. Slowly, indifference settled over us like a spell, dulling our senses, until being overlooked felt as natural as breathing - just another rhythm in the endless, indifferent pulse of the hospital around us.

By the fifth week, the days had blurred into a muted, unchanging rhythm, like a story unfolding in soft focus, the details slipping by unnoticed. I watched it all with my eyes half-closed, lulled by the routine. But that week, something changed - a tug, a sudden, sharp pull that yanked my eyes open, forcing me to see it all with unsettling clarity.

Monday's rounds brought us to a five-year-old boy, small and frail, with pain etched into his face that felt too heavy for his tiny frame. In a *Paediatric* ward, a sick child wasn't unusual, but this room carried a strange, chilly quiet that clung to the air, the kind that makes you shiver despite the warmth. He waited for his *bone marrow biopsy* results, the doctors murmuring their fears - *leukaemia, lymphoma* - and the room seemed to absorb the dread, every inch of it heavy and shadowed. Other rooms housed sound; though sick, the children were loud, and their parents darted around them unless the child was asleep. But here, the air was still, as if laughter had been banished. The boy barely glanced up, his gaze fixed to the TV, immune to the team's jokes that fell into silence. Even now, I can't recall a single social smile from that room, just an emptiness that sadness alone couldn't explain.

Tuesday morning, I clocked in early, arriving at the hospital at 7:45 to catch the pre-rounds. By 8:33 - give or take a heartbeat - the attending's phone chimed, its soft ding cutting through the resident presenting her patient's updates. The results were in. I watched as his expression shifted. The resident paused, holding her flowing word gates. A flicker of urgency lit up in his eyes as he pulled up the five-year-old's patient details. We still had five rooms to visit before this patient, but something in him refused to wait. The residents murmured about timing, but he waved them off, intent. We moved swiftly, each step carrying us closer to the room, the answer waiting in black and white: No signs of *Malignancy*. No cancer. What remained was a possibility of *Kawasaki*.

I barely remember the seconds that followed - the attending asked for the room number, and then, without a single thought, we were off, sprinting through the maze of wards. The attending was taking large strides, and at some point, he started running, the sound echoing around us like a heartbeat. By the time we stumbled into the room, breathless, the doctor managed to steady himself just enough to get the words out: it wasn't cancer.

Relief washed over the family. And that's when I saw it: the room, lifeless and colourless just yesterday, seemed to pulse with a new warmth, colours unfurling like a sunrise crept over the walls. It was as if the air had been filled with light and fragrance, the hope so tangible, it felt like you could reach out and touch it. I stood there, stunned, behind the whole team, the space transforming before my eyes, as if life itself had returned to the room. I could feel as though the ground had softened beneath me, moulding into a hollow where my feet had pressed, like the room itself had anchored me there, unwilling to let me drift from the weight of that moment.

We stayed in the room as the team explained the diagnosis to the family, their voices soft and careful. I stayed silent, rooted to the spot, still stunned by the colours and warmth that had bloomed around us. I couldn't shake the feeling that yesterday, I'd missed something, that vibrancy of this room had been invisible to me until now. Today I could see it, smell it, even palpate it - the air felt richer, tinged with a fragrance I couldn't name. The tears streaming down every face in the room left my legs weak, and all I could do was lean against the wall, observing. That moment carved itself into my memory, etched deep, like an image that would never fade.

Kawasaki isn't supposed to be a gentle diagnosis. Normally, it arrives like a storm cloud, casting a dark, lingering shadow over the child's health. The kind of diagnosis that drains colour from parents' faces, leaving them in shades of fear and helplessness. But here in this tiny, muted room, *Kawasaki* transformed into something almost fairy-like, a whimsical stroke of fate that brought smiles and sounds instead of sorrow. Against all odds, it was the bright thread woven into a rather dark tapestry, a rare moment when the word itself felt lighter, shimmering, as if it had a soft glow - something magical that turned dread into hope. The kind of miracle that makes you believe, if only for a second, that even diagnoses can be charmed.

Later, the doctor explained himself, his voice steady but softened by the relief still radiating through him. "I couldn't let them suffer a moment longer," he said, his eyes holding a quiet intensity, as if he, too, was only beginning to understand the gravity of what he'd done. The truth of it landed heavily and exhilaratingly in the quiet space between his words. As he spoke, something settled over all of us in the ward lobby - a sense of wonder, an understanding that what we'd just witnessed was more than medicine. It was life, saved in the gentlest way, like pulling someone back from the edge of a cliff without ever knowing they were about to fall.

The phrase "doctors save lives" hit me for the first time. It didn't feel like something we'd heard in a lecture or textbook. It had shape, texture, a realness that settled into my chest and warmed my bones. It was as though, in that instant, something invisible and shimmering had wrapped around all of us in the room, a shared breath of relief that swelled into our chests, like a little bit of magical glitter was swirling within.

In that fleeting silence, I could feel it - an unspoken understanding passing among us, a current of pride, joy, and awe all tangled together. The family's tears were mingled with smiles, soft but real, felt like a rare gift. Standing there, I realised I'd witnessed something magical. Something that wouldn't easily fade. I felt what it truly meant to heal, not just in the clinical sense but in the quiet, indescribable way a heart heals when it's been given back hope. And as we left the room, that glow lingered, a light we carried with us. A reminder that sometimes, amidst all the chaos and uncertainty, there is a moment where medicine feels like magic.

THE POWER OF ESTABLISHING RAPPORT

Dr Meharish Ambatt

Aspiring surgeons often worry about the dexterity of their hands and the precision of their skills. They also carry the weight of ensuring the success of the procedures they may one day perform.

However, being a good surgeon isn't limited to the skill of performing the surgery alone, but rather goes above and beyond. A lot of our expertise and scope of care extends further into the way we interact with our patients and their families, *pre-* and *post-operatively*. This influences the quality of the care they receive and ultimately the patient outcome.

In a teaching hospital, *residents* are the ground team who interact with patients on a day-to-day basis and spend the most time with them throughout their stay (other than the nursing team, of course). As residents, we see inpatients (patients admitted inside the hospital) daily or sometimes even more than once a day by visiting them during rounds. Thereby, we watch their progress or deterioration to the most minute detail and get the honour of establishing a meaningful rapport along the way. By knowing them so closely and detecting minor changes, we're also able to make timely decisions that improve their care significantly.

One encounter has been particularly striking for me. I once had a patient who was an elderly man suffering from *cholecystitis* (inflammation of the gallbladder) and was scheduled to undergo a *laparoscopic cholecystectomy* (removal of the gallbladder).

Throughout the days leading up to his surgery, I'd noticed that he'd often be accompanied by his children, who loved him dearly.

This was evident in their efforts to research his condition and the concerns and questions they would express regarding his day-to-day progress and further management options.

Patient education and counselling, both of which are integral aspects of our training, must often be tailored to the background and expectations of the patient. While patients with minimal literacy may require the breaking down of information into simplified examples, someone who's well-educated may have higher expectations regarding the intricate details of the procedure. To deliver the information in an individualised manner is an art and a skill in its own right.

As my current patient's family often requested finer details, I used to spend extra time with them trying to explain the procedure, often using true anatomical diagrams and drawing on them to explain every step of the procedure, along with expected complications. However, I did not realise the extent of the impression I was forming or the rapport I'd been building through this process until the day they asked me, "So, who will be performing the surgery?"

A question I had been all too familiar with throughout my journey. Patients usually express concerns and queries about the surgeon because they would prefer to know the expertise, skill, or position of the surgeon. More often than not, they're hoping to hear that someone at the highest position, who has done the procedure a few hundred times, will be doing their surgery, as that's what convinces them that they're truly in safe hands.

As is our hospital protocol, I informed them that the surgical team for any particular day will depend on the schedule, which will definitely include a senior surgeon. "However," I added reassuringly, "I would be around on the day, and if I'm not engaged in any other activity as per the distribution of work, I'll be attending the surgery as well." Their response, however, was truly unexpected for me and touched me in a way that I'll cherish forever.

"We would be happy if you're the one who'll be performing the surgery," they'd told me that memorable day. "You're the one whom we've been seeing every day. You're the one who has been communicating with us, explaining everything, preparing us mentally and so on. You're the one we know and trust to do the surgery." I was taken aback by the amount of trust and confidence they placed in me, primarily due to the rapport that I'd built along the way.

At this point in my journey, I was already a senior resident who had done my fair share of *cholecystectomies* as needed for my level and was confident to perform the same for my patient. But what surprised me was that while his family knew I was a trainee, they did not know my exact level of training, and neither did they seem to want to know how many successful cholecystectomies I had performed, or how many years of experience I had behind me. They did not seem to care about my college scores or *residency* rankings - things all medical trainees give undue importance to.

From the moment we decide to pursue medicine, we begin to judge ourselves, our potential, and our skills by our test scores, the number of cases we've seen, the number of surgeries we've done, or the number of certificates we've collected. We assume that our success in the field would depend strictly on our educational background or the labels of our positions.

However, what the patients are really looking for in their surgeon is the healing touch and the human connection. Naturally, they find it easier to trust and rely on a surgeon who has taken the time and effort to see them as human beings, addressing their concerns, alleviating their fears, and comforting them in their distress. None of these expectations depends on the number of degrees or level of seniority. But rather, at the heart of it all is a simple yet profound truth: a sense of humanity.

In the increasingly competitive field of medical education and training, it's all too easy to put the focus solely on the numbers. But above and beyond numbers, the impact we create and the ripples we make in our communities come from the lives we've touched and the trust we've acquired with our diligent and compassionate services. When we start establishing our practice as healthcare professionals, we can attain better access to patients via word-of-mouth recommendations by those who are satisfied with our care in a better way than by being known for our academic certifications or the length of our resumes alone.

To continuously improve as healthcare providers, we must pause and ask ourselves, "What have I done to establish a connection with my patient today - to treat them as a living, breathing human being with fears and concerns, rather than just another case to jot down in my logbook?"

More importantly, "Would I as a patient like to be treated the way I treat my patients? Would I like for a friend or family member of mine to be treated this way?" If the answer is negative, perhaps we can reflect on what steps we can take to change that answer to a resounding "Yes!" After all, at the heart of our profession is patient satisfaction. Everything else is secondary and follows suit accordingly.

THE UNFORGETTABLE DOCTOR'S GIFT

Dr Lekshmi Nath

As I walked into the hospital that crisp morning, the hospital doors opened, welcoming me into another day of unknown challenges. The weight of responsibility pressed on my shoulders as it always did, but something in the air felt different - an unspoken urgency, a day that would carve itself into my memory forever.

As an *obstetrician*, each day, I witness the miracle of life and the fragility that comes with it. That day, however, was destined to be different.

I had just finished reviewing my schedule when a nurse rushed in, her face pale. "Doctor, we are ready." I grabbed my coat and hurried to the operating theatre. The sight that greeted me was one of controlled chaos. Nurses and doctors were working frantically around the patient who lay on the bed, her face contorted in pain.

Anjali had been my patient for several years. Previously, I had performed surgery on her to remove *fibroids* from her uterus. Fibroids are usually *benign* structures that abnormally grow in and around the uterus. One of their complications can be infertility. After having undergone the surgery, she was able to become pregnant soon and came to me for her check-ups.

At twenty-two weeks of her pregnancy, however, we had to place a stitch for her as her birth canal was short, and she was at risk of losing the baby anytime. She was then hospitalised until thirty-six weeks. For almost three months, she was on bed rest with elevation of her legs to provide support and avoid the loss of her unborn child. Her perseverance and trust in the process were truly remarkable.

As a case of high-risk pregnancy, we prepared for a C-section, knowing that every second counted. The operating room was a blur of movement and sound, but amidst the chaos, there was a strange sense of calmness within me. I had done this countless times, yet each time felt just as critical. One of the nurses briefed me about her condition. I took a deep breath, summoning all the years of training and experience I had. "Please, save my baby," she whispered. I nodded, feeling the gravity of her words.

The surgery began, and I could feel the tension in the room. My focus was razor-sharp. As she dozed off under *anaesthesia*, we worked, and the minutes felt like hours. Finally, we heard the sound we had all been waiting for - the cry of a newborn. It was weak but unmistakable. We had delivered a baby girl. The *neonatology* team took over, working quickly to stabilise the tiny infant. I turned my attention back to my patient, ensuring she was stable. Once I was certain she was out of immediate danger, I allowed myself a moment of relief.

I stepped out of the operating theatre. Anjali's mother stood beside the door, with tears streaming down her face. "Doctor," she said, her voice choking with emotion, "thank you for saving my daughter and her baby." I smiled, feeling a lump in my throat. "She's a fighter, just like her mother."

Later, when the baby's birth certificate arrived, there it was in official print - "Lekshmi Nath."

I was taken aback and deeply touched. "That's a beautiful name," I said, my voice barely above a whisper. At that moment, I felt a profound connection to this family. I had been given the honour of being part of their story, a story of hope and resilience.

Baby Lekshmi's journey was just beginning, but I knew she had the strength of her mother and the love of her family to see her through. Her name, a symbol of hope and gratitude, was a reminder that every life we touch as doctors leaves an indelible mark.

As I left the hospital that evening, the sky painted in hues of twilight, I felt a profound sense of fulfilment. I had done my duty, but more than that, I had witnessed a miracle - a miracle born from the convergence of hope, trust, and relentless perseverance. Their unwavering trust in me and the sacrifice she and her family made were humbling reminders of the profound responsibility that comes with being a doctor.

Reflecting on the day's events, I realised that medicine is not just about treatments and procedures; it is about forging deep connections and being present in the most intimate moments of people's lives. Walking to my car, I felt a renewed sense of purpose. As the stars began to emerge in the night sky, I knew that the story of this patient and her daughter would stay with me forever, inspiring me to continue my journey with compassion and dedication.

THE CROCHETED CONNECTION

Dr Sumaiyya Shersad

As a family doctor working in a small city in England, I often feel the weight of responsibility of caring for a community with diverse healthcare needs. I strive to make people feel heard and understood, but with the complex nature of chronic health conditions, some days it can be difficult to know whether I'm making a difference at all. One patient, in particular, has etched herself into my heart: Mrs Eleanor Matthews, a woman in her late sixties with a myriad of disabling health problems and resultant *chronic* pain.

She had been a regular visitor to my office over the past year; each appointment bearing testament to her struggle with pain and her fight to find some semblance of normalcy. Her arthritic hands and frail body bore the weight of countless battles fought silently. More than once, she had confided in me her darkest thoughts, that life no longer felt worth living.

The weight of the *Hippocratic Oath* rests heavily on my shoulders each day, a constant reminder of my duty to ease suffering and uphold the sanctity of life. As such, I always made it a point to listen to her with compassion, offering words of encouragement and hope. I would spend extra time with her, adjusting medications, suggesting new therapies, and simply being a comforting presence. We shared many conversations about life and the importance of finding joy in the smallest of things.

One of those regular appointments, Eleanor shuffled in, her face etched with familiar lines of pain. That day, however, there was something different in her eyes – a glimmer of resolve. After discussing her current treatment plan and making sure she had everything she needed, she reached into her cloth tote.

"I made this," she said, her voice quivering with a mix of pride and anticipation. She pulled out a beautiful white crocheted bag, its delicate patterns a testament to the countless hours she had spent crafting it. "This is for you because you gave me hope when I was at my lowest."

I was choked with emotion, knowing the pain she endured daily, and the immense effort it must have taken her to create such a beautiful piece. The intricacy of the stitches, the care in each loop - it was a labour of love and gratitude that transcended words.

As I took the bag in my hands, the weight of her struggle and my own role in her journey overwhelmed me. With tear-filled eyes, I looked at Eleanor, who was watching me with a soft, understanding smile.

"Eleanor, this is... I don't know what to say," I said, my voice thick with emotion. "This means more to me than you can ever know." She reached out and gently clasped my hand with her fingers. "You've done so much more for me than just treating my ailments. You listened when I thought no one cared, and you gave me hope when I had none. This bag is just a small token of my appreciation."

In that moment, the sterile walls of the office seemed to fade away, replaced by a profound connection between two souls. It wasn't just about the physical healing; it was about the emotional support I had provided, the lifeline extended to her time and time again.

I hugged her gently, careful not to cause her pain. "Thank you. This is the most precious gift I've ever received."

As she left the office, I sat quietly for a moment, clutching the crocheted bag to my chest. I realised that being a doctor is not just about prescribing medicine or diagnosing ailments; it is about the human connections, the empathy, and the hope that can be kindled even in the darkest of times.

That day, as I left the practice, Eleanor's gift reminded me why I had chosen this path in the first place. It is for moments like these - for the lives touched, the hopes restored, and the silent battles fought together. And with that thought, I stepped out, carrying with me a heart full of gratitude and a beautiful white crocheted bag.

TREATMENT WITH COMPASSION

Dr Faatimah Maryam Muzammil

As we all step into the medical world, at some point, we take an adapted version of the *Hippocratic Oath*. To an onlooker, it might be words strung together, but for doctors, it is a promise of a lifetime.

To me, the essence of medicine is best understood by this quote written by Hippocrates: "Wherever the art of medicine is loved, there is a love of humanity."

Throughout our medical journey, we spend gruelling years learning and relearning facts, mnemonics, and patient care. It is expected that doctors eventually become desensitised to most disease presentations. While this approach may help an individual to work objectively for the patient, it hinders a deeper understanding of problems and creates roadblocks in providing optimum patient-centric care. I realised this better when I encountered a patient who reminded me of the beauty of this profession.

As I walked into the corridors of the *Cardiology* ward, I entered the room of a fifty-six-year-old man named Mr A. He was seated comfortably on the bed and was smiling from ear to ear. As I entered and greeted him, he seemed enthusiastic and well. As I continued to ask him questions, his *history* revealed a *chief complaint* of chest pain. Before coming to our emergency, he had presented to another clinic where he complained of *epigastric pain* and was discharged home on medicines for acidity. He went back to another clinic two days later with similar complaints and was again dismissed.

Finally, he visited our emergency department for increasing and worsening pain. Although his *ECG* was normal, his blood tests indicated that something sinister could have been causing his chest pain. It was a *myocardial infarction*, or in simple words, he was having a heart attack! He was then rushed for treatment to save his life, as every passing second was precious to prevent further damage to his failing heart.

As he narrated his story, I couldn't help but notice his smile and comforting demeanour. At the end of the *history*, when we asked him permission to *examine* his chest and *auscultate*, he gladly agreed. He then told us, "If I don't let you, as students, examine me, how will you all become good doctors? I want to be a source of learning for you."

We finally wished him health and bid him adieu. As we were walking out, he wished us the best of luck in our medical careers and gave us so many prayers. I was truly inspired by his sincere desire for us to learn and do better. In our medical journey, we read thousands of resources, but one of the best teachers for all of us is our patients. Their presentations and diagnostic challenges help us practically apply our knowledge, and their unique experiences become stories we use to teach our juniors.

Mr A not only taught me the knowledge I needed in the cardiovascular unit, but he also taught me a much greater lesson of compassion. Although he was a patient in our healthcare facility, he displayed such kindness to us that I felt a sense of contentment having the chance to be involved in his care. His smile was a testament to the fact that gestures that spread happiness will always be remembered for a long time.

As doctors, we must always treat our patients with compassion and grace. They come to us in some of the most frightening and vulnerable moments of their lives, filled with questions and fears. It is both our responsibility and our privilege to care for them in the best way possible. Every patient deserves to be treated with the highest level of respect, empathy, and unwavering dedication.

MOTHER, SON AND PRIVILEGE

Dr Raabeah Fatma Jafri

When I started my *clinical* rotations as an undergraduate medical student, I developed a strange hyper-fixation. After returning home every day, I would open my diary and write down every single thing that happened that day, from the detailed *histories* I took from my patients to the jokes I made with my friends. Every. Single. Day. Some days, it would even take hours owing to the minute details and significant events of the placement. Although this habit of mine may seem random, bear this in mind as it shall soon become relevant.

After all, it's a small world out there. We see and meet people every day. Each one of these interactions has an impact on us. Whether positive or negative, conscious or subconscious, every encounter leaves its mark.

The day I'm about to recount was not particularly remarkable, yet some memories tend to linger. I was a third-year medical student in my *OBGYN* rotation. It was sometime in June (I remember because I wrote it in my diary). My colleague and I had just taken a history in the *labour* suite from a young Arab woman in her thirties who was expecting the arrival of her third child. She was in the early stages of labour and not in the most comfortable state. Regardless, she wore an incredibly welcoming smile. She answered our questions extensively despite a significant language barrier and the fact that we were quite slow and hesitant as we were still new to the process.

Her pregnancy was considered high-risk compared to her previous two. Nevertheless, our conversation with her was refreshing, and it was amazing to see how excited she was to meet her baby boy!

Later, we discussed our history with our supervising doctor and moved on. (Of course, I wrote everything down in my diary that afternoon.) Unfortunately, we were not able to be present at her delivery as we had been posted in a different section for the rest of the week. Being a medical student often means that we don't really stay in one department for more than a month (high turnover, if you will). This means that we see a lot of patients either for the first or last time. This also means that we only have thirty minutes, if not less, to build rapport with a patient that we will most likely never see again. Although we're enormously grateful for the multiple opportunities to see so many patients, the sadness creeps in on realising that we may not see them again.

Fast forward to a couple of months, when I was a fourth-year medical student in the outpatient *Paediatric* Surgery department. Again, it wasn't a particularly eventful day; most of the patients were infants being brought for *pre-operative* check-ups. One of the patients who came in was a four-month-old baby boy brought by his father. He was adorable, with big brown eyes and chubby cheeks. His mother entered the clinic room a couple of minutes later, and there was no doubt that I had seen that very smile before. I wasn't sure who she was or how I knew her, but there was an air of familiarity. I listened intently as the doctor asked the parents for details about the birth of the baby.

That day, upon returning home, I rummaged through my diary full of seemingly mundane histories and matched the history about the baby boy to the history I had taken from his mother about four months ago. The *gestational* age, the date of birth, the mode of delivery, and the *antenatal* history - it was a perfect match!

There was no doubt it was the same patient, that the woman I found familiar was the mother I had met during her third delivery.

Who would have thought that, four months later, in an entirely different setting, we would meet again! What a relief to know that she had given birth to a healthy baby boy. What a relief to know that she was alive and well, smiling as she always did. What a relief to know that the blessing she had been so excited for was sitting in her lap. All the risks, tests, contractions – it was all worth it!

I had absolutely no role in the care of this patient, but this experience gave me a taste of the medical profession - to see your patient in discomfort and distress, and having the privilege to ease their pain is a blessing indeed. It is a privilege to see them again in a better state of health and happiness. It is a privilege to not just make them better physically, but also to make them feel better mentally and emotionally.

I wasn't entirely sure what I felt that day, but it was a monumental day in my life that I wish to never forget.

Now, as a medical intern, when I look back at my medical student self, I realise that, yes, that was indeed one of the many beautiful gifts of my profession. It is the blessing of knowledge, understanding, the art of listening, and the fortune of witnessing such precious moments of people's lives. A privilege that keeps so many of us going despite the multiple hurdles in our path. It moulds us into who we are today and will be in the future. *Alhamdulillah* (All thanks and praise be to God).

THE FIRST CRANIAL NERVE

Dr Reema

The *olfactory nerve*, also known as the first *cranial nerve*, governs our sense of smell, a peculiar ability that deeply influences our daily experiences. As someone with a particularly sensitive nose, I've always made an effort to ensure I smelled pleasant by using moisturisers, deodorants, and dousing myself with perfumes. Whenever I encountered unpleasant odours, be it putrid, fishy, or otherwise repulsive, I instinctively blocked my nose, opting instead to breathe through my mouth. To me, smelling good was more than a habit; it was a part of my self-expression and comfort. However, during my medical student years, a memorable encounter taught me that not everyone has the privilege of controlling what they can and cannot smell.

It happened in a breast clinic, a setting I eagerly looked forward to. As a medical student, I relished the opportunity to learn through hands-on experience, and this clinic was the perfect setting to hone my skills in *physical examination* through *palpation.* I encountered a myriad of cases ranging from mobile *fibroadenomas*, fixed *axillary* masses, *gynaecomastia* in male patients, post-*mastectomy seromas*, each a valuable learning opportunity to develop my diagnostic acumen and tactile skills.

As the clinic was nearing its end, a patient in her early forties walked in. She avoided eye contact, staring at the floor, and wore a thick cardigan that she kept wrapping over her chest, despite the scorching 38°C heat outside. Her demeanour was subdued, almost apologetic. I overheard the doctor discussing the need to provide the patient with extra *gauze* and *incontinence pads*, though I didn't immediately understand why.

The patient hesitated. It was time for her *examination.* As I was reaching to draw the curtains around the bed to ensure privacy, she turned to me and said softly, "I'm terribly sorry, I smell bad. Please wear a mask." Her words caught me off guard, and I quickly reassured her, saying I didn't notice any smell and that it was completely fine. I wanted to put her at ease, but I didn't yet understand the gravity of her situation. As the patient removed her sweater and exposed her chest, I finally understood. Her left breast was obscured by a *fungating* mass that had completely distorted its shape. The mass extended down to occupy the entire breast. It was friable, bleeding with even the slightest touch, and oozing *necrotic* fluid.

And then there was the smell, the unmistakable, pungent odour of *necrotic* tissue.

A surgical *resident* stepped forward, assisting the patient with remarkable compassion and care. She gently wiped the blood dripping from the breast, cleaned the necrotic areas, and comforted the patient, who repeatedly apologised, saying, "I'm so sorry for making this room stink. I'm sorry for making you change my dressing."

As I stood nearby, I felt helpless and heartbroken, knowing that beyond dressing changes, there was little we could do for her to change her reality. Yet, the *resident*'s approach was a masterclass in empathy and kindness. She continuously reassured the patient, reminding her that none of this was her fault.

Inspired by her example, I decided to step forward. I assisted with the dressing changes, handing the resident fresh gauze and disposing off the soiled ones. My role was small, almost insignificant, but it felt essential to show the patient that we were all there for her, not as passive, detached observers, but as active participants and caregivers united in solidarity. I realised that for her, this was not just a moment of discomfort - it was her everyday reality.

Through her tears, the patient revealed the impact of her condition on her life. She hadn't seen friends in months, fearing judgement. She lived alone, isolated, and the smell from her breast had overwhelmed her to the point that she could no longer eat properly. Her sense of smell had dulled, leaving her trapped with the relentless odour of *necrosis.*

After she left, the smell lingered in the room, a haunting reminder of her reality. I never saw her again, but I continue to hope for the best for her.

This encounter was a moment of introspection for me. Here I was, someone who obsessively curated my own sensory experiences, faced with the reality of someone who had no control over hers. I realised how much I had taken simple things like smelling good or feeling confident in social settings for granted. For this patient, no amount of effort could mask the reality of her condition.

This experience also deepened my resolve as an aspiring surgeon. It reminded me that while medicine has made incredible strides, there are still countless diseases and conditions that demand more effective treatments and compassionate care. The resident's approach to the patient was a powerful lesson: caregiving isn't just about addressing physical symptoms; it's about seeing the person behind the condition, offering them dignity and humanity in their most vulnerable moments.

From that day on, I carried with me the lessons I learned in that clinic, not just about clinical *examination*, but about the essence of empathy and solidarity. Medicine is not just a science; it is a deeply human endeavour. It requires us to step beyond our own comfort, to breathe in the reality of others, and to offer care that heals not only the body but also the spirit.

CAT PICTURES AND BLOOD CANCER

Tiba Aldelaimi

A possibility of cancer.

This is what the current patient presents with. She is sitting with her hands on her lap, observing the picture of a cat wearing a little white coat on the otherwise bare wall. The doctor is in luck as he does not have to discuss with her this possibility, nor is he able to, as he is preoccupied. New to the electronic system in this hospital, his eyes make many trips between the keyboard and monitor as he is still typing up the last patient's notes with a single finger. She and I have been sitting for what feels like the past forty-five minutes in this cold office. People usually try to engage him in small talk to fill the silence of his trips, but inevitably resort to their phones until he is done. I am trying not to doze off sitting behind the doctor, and she is sitting in front of him, still silent, sometimes staring at the almost bare wall or looking at her hands in her lap. The seconds and clicks go by, and all three of us age to the faint sounds of the keyboard.

Once cancer is part of the process, the steady stream of referrals and procedures flows fast. I get to see her again in a few days. She is now facing the bare wall of the procedure room, lying down on her side in a polyester gown with a small square of skin over the back of her hip bone exposed and sanitised. There's a *pathologist* with his trainees and three nurses, all on the side of the room facing away from her. I wonder if she has realised, somewhere deep down, that this is the furthest thing from a routine check-up. I am standing at the door, steeling my nerves to ask her if I may be present for her *bone marrow aspiration.* Minutes ago, my doctor had advised me against asking for permission. I had not spoken to her before, and if I cared about observing this procedure, he said, I should not risk allowing her to refuse me, and, with so many people already in the room, what would one more mean?

When I ask her for permission, she smiles, quietly says yes, says of course, says that I am a part of the team. And so, I walk further in and interrupt the swath of beige paint in front of her. From here, I have a full view of her and everyone else in this room behind her. I had not seen a bone marrow aspiration before, but I read that this procedure would include a hollow needle. I did not realise it would be one so large that it glints under the bright fluorescents of the ceiling. This is inserted into the bone, and an amount is taken to be prepared and studied. And now the doctor walks up behind her, puts the large, shiny needle into her hip bone, and pulls.

The core of many people's anxiety around both healthcare and death is a fear of suffering. From where I am standing, I see why. I watch how her eyebrows scrunch, how her mouth thins into a line; the pain on her face is obvious, and because she is holding her breath, silent. I understand why everyone else had stood behind her. She looks up at me, and I do not - cannot - look away. When he is done, he hands the sample to the pathologist in the corner, and he and the students start preparing it. A nurse comes forward to press on her wound and tells the woman she 'did so well' and 'it's all over now.' The students whisper to the pathologist what cells they identify, and their descriptions are as quiet as the underlying disease is obvious. A curtain of dread encompassing the procedure room is a difficult thing to ignore.

The weight of certainty is heavy. Being forced to face the body's limited mortality is an unsettling experience. The doctor assures the woman that 'everything is fine,' 'there's nothing to worry about,' and that he is 'just taking a sample to check' and tells me we are leaving. But I do not want to leave before I thank her. I was still standing in front of her, and we had started making small talk at some point. I do not know if I am providing a much-needed distraction or if I am naively burdening the woman with these pleasantries. In a situation like this, small talk was the only skill I could rely on: I was building up to expressing 'thank you.' The doctor's head pokes in from behind the door, and he is calling me to get out and leave her to rest. And the only way I know to briskly express my gratitude for the experience she had allowed me to be part of is to hand her her phone. She declines it and holds my hand instead.

I never saw her after that. It strikes me how she was always by herself. I wonder if she went through the treatment options alone, too. I wonder if she will remember the cat picture on the wall or the colour of the paint. I still see the doctor sometimes. I wonder if he types any faster. I wonder if the empathy in my assigned lectures translates just as clumsily in real life. I wonder if I will still have empathy with myself in my clinical years when I don't have any procedures to see for the first time again, and when my shift is eight hours long, and I can't take breaks in between appointments. Bones will break, and tumours will grow, and large, shiny needles will be needed at every age. I will meet more people like her, and by the end of all of this, I hope I don't wonder whether I made a difference.

ANATOMY OF BECOMING

Dr Amna Ibrahim Zaidan

"Two roads diverged in a wood, and I – I took the one less travelled by, and that has made all the difference." - Robert Frost

Our beginning was a passion for saving lives. In medical school, it was a curiosity to learn. In *clinical* rotations, it was making someone's reality better than how it is.

Right now, I know it's much more than that.

About Our Role Models

In one of my *emergency* rotations as a medical student, I had a hard time adjusting to the fast-paced environment and keeping up with all the doctors. It was a stressful, unsettling setting with nurses running around suddenly, patients vomiting in hallways, screams heard from inside closed curtains, children crying, and me, standing in the middle of that. However, being a self-challenging individual, I wanted to be involved.

That's when I saw the most colourful running shoes paired with navy scrubs - an emergency medicine consultant who asked me if I had ever done a *urinary catheterisation* before. He was like an Avengers character, at least to me. He not only involved me and my colleagues in patient care but also gave us teaching sessions regarding the cases we encountered. I felt like I was where I belonged and where I needed to be. I was lucky to have been there when he was around. I ambitiously wish that all doctors would become like that. We wouldn't have a toxic work environment, and each team member would be valued.

Now, let's take a step back. When we're asked about who we look up to as medical students or interns, we tend to think of medical professionals or professors we encountered. But what about the people closest to us? The ones who, without their support, we wouldn't be where we are right now. Personally, I would not be able to see the end of my medical school graduation if it weren't for the support of my parents and my whole family, my backbone. Being there for me in my crying sessions before exams. Telling me it was okay when it wasn't, so I would only focus on studying, not on tuition fees. Fighting alongside me against every adversity that comes my way.

Those are the unseen role models that should come up before anyone else. I should be saying this more often: Mama, Baba, I wouldn't be here without you. Thank you, always.

Being Humble is Not Just Noble

"Medicine is a noble profession."

We hear this a lot. But what does it really mean? I will tell you what it doesn't mean: Arrogance. Getting a medical degree and going through the toughest major and sacrifices in social life is definitely commendable, as it is a dream turned into reality. But this does not qualify a doctor to become superior to anyone else, especially to their patients.

A patient is someone whom we'll meet for the first time, just like any other person. They will develop a first impression and judge you based on your appearance and attitude. But, there's a significant difference between other people you meet and patients: *Vulnerability*.

Patients are not there because they want to; they are there because they need to. They were given the option to choose any doctor out there, and yet they chose you. They chose to trust you. Being honest and open about their discomforts or the 'abnormalities' they are going through is a sensitive conversation to get into. It's what we usually hide from the closest people to us, and yet, when we're in a doctor's office, we are expected to be truthful and answer uncomfortable questions by trusting that stranger wearing a white coat sitting in front of us, staring at a computer screen.

What a "Good Doctor" Looks Like

The wardrobe consists of either scrubs or formal, casual attire under a crisp, ironed white coat. Scent is ethanol with a hint of citrus. A well-kept hijab on top or a neat hairdo. A doctor is passing by. Squared shoulders and a proper soldier's march down the hospital hallway. A welcoming smile and nod to the patients waiting outside before entering the office. This is a scenario describing a perfect start to the day. Remembering that the attitude a doctor reflects is the first thing a patient notices will allow you to comfort anxious hearts. And keeping in mind that you are not too good for a task, a case, or a patient will ground you morally. Getting *intravenous (IV)* access yourself from a patient because the nurses are busy is okay. Managing flu cases and sick leave requests all day is okay. A confused, scared patient not understanding their diagnosis, even though you're explaining it for the fifth time, is okay.

Is Empathy Still Alive?

While I was posted as a fifth-year medical student in the *Emergency Department*, a nurse asked me to translate to a patient that she needed to wear adult diapers to urinate. While relaying that message to the patient, I realised that my job there was to actually convince the patient. She refused both *urinary catheterisation* and adult diapers adamantly. The nurse's justification was that the patient was not allowed to go to the bathroom alone, as she is currently recovering from *hypoglycaemia* and she is at high risk of fainting, which was her main symptom when she first came to the Emergency Department.

Being a free-spirited medical student with lots of time on my hands, I listened to the patient, empathised with her, and thoroughly explained to her the risks and benefits. However, I secretly felt it was vague that this was the sole management option. Finally, she said she'll think about it when I told the nurses that, with a feeling of achievement, they started laughing in front of the patient. To them, she was one of many patients, and they had more work to do than wait for her to decide. The doctor finally came in through the curtain, and I sighed with relief. He told the nurse, "If you were in her place, would you want to wear a diaper and urinate in it?" He explained that it's natural to feel humiliated and undignified if one were in her place. Instead, he said she could use a *commode chair*, to which the patient agreed.

This was a eureka moment for me. While being distracted by the task given to me by the nurses to convince the patient, I became apathetic. It was a case to me, not a patient anymore. When sympathy is numb inside us, we no longer believe the pain of the patient.

Hospitals, especially emergency departments, are unfamiliar to most patients. They don't come to the emergency department daily like us. They are not used to hearing a son wailing outside in the hallway after his mother died in front of him due to a *cardiac arrest*. They have not seen parents stand there feeling powerless, watching their daughter with *cerebral palsy* take her last breaths. They have not seen a husband break down in tears while embracing his wife's cold, blue, dead body. They just want to get out of there as soon as possible, while those who lost their loved ones want to stay there for as long as possible.

For those who have seen more than they should

News flash: Doctors can get sick, too. What doctors see in hospitals is traumatising enough for them to develop *panic disorders* and *post-traumatic stress disorders*. Not to mention that health professionals are known to be at high risk of *depression* and burnout. For our dear colleagues and our fellow doctors, who deserve recognition for their sacrifices and for continuing this journey despite all its difficulties, *You are your number one priority*.

No flu that you catch from a patient can be compared to the agony of a depressive episode that resulted from bottling up emotions or several burnouts. Apathy can affect patient care and make you hate your job. We need to recognise our own damage before we see the wounds on other people. You can't pour from an empty cup.

Acknowledging Mess-Ups

When I was posted in *Obstetrics and Gynaecology (OBGYN)* emergency, there was one *consultant* OBGYN doctor assigned to many beds on a busy Friday. And then there was I, a fifth-year medical student. The doctor seemed extremely stressed out while filling out documents and seeing patients. Amidst all this, there was a pregnant patient who came complaining of vaginal bleeding. Upon undergoing an *ultrasound* scan, it was apparent that she had a *missed miscarriage*.

After confirming the miscarriage by completing the scan, the doctor was about to leave. That's when the patient asked her, "How is my baby?" to which the doctor replied in an irritated tone, "What baby? There's no baby!" Needless to mention, the patient was shocked and began crying sorrowfully. An hour later, however, the doctor came back and apologised to her.

What I learned from that encounter is that no matter how busy we can be, patients will only understand their pain. They don't have the luxury of understanding their doctor while they are in their most vulnerable state. We, as doctors, are merely human. We are bound to make mistakes, which makes us human. What we can do about it in a hospital setting is acknowledge our mistake and take responsibility for it because we are not divine; we're merely human beings. That must always humble us.

When patients come to us with their eyes in need and plead for our help with nervousness, trying their best not to show their fear, we must not ridicule, demean, or underestimate their pain. We all have different levels of tolerance. Our job is not just to understand diseases but to understand that there are humans just like us who are suffering because of those diseases.

We will definitely face difficult patients who might ruin our day with rude remarks, or they might shout or undervalue all our efforts in helping them. The obvious answer in such cases is to remain professional and to manoeuvre our way out of it somehow and resolve the situation. But the not-so-talked-about question is: *What about us?* "Perfectionism" might be one of our qualities, but "Perfect" is not an adjective we associate with. We will get hurt, upset, frustrated, and angry. Those emotions need to be unleashed somewhere.

Self-expression doesn't come easily to us since we're either in a position where we must care for people who depend on us to get better, or we are in a competitive work environment. An environment where we must never show our weaknesses, or else they will be taken advantage of.

We have family and we have friends, and maybe even strangers, to confide in. A listening ear is just what we need sometimes. And I mean, just a listening ear, none of the "If you're so stressed out, then why don't you just quit?" or "You chose to pursue medicine." comments. You don't usually hear those scolding remarks from colleagues because they feel your pain (most of them, at least).

An Office Job

Most of a doctor's work in this modern urban world has become administrative. Doctors spend more time charting and finishing administrative work rather than spending that time understanding their patients better by indulging in conversation and thoroughly interviewing them. Being in hospitals and health centres during my time as a medical student and *intern* now, I have observed how many doctors miss a detail or two due to rushing the interview in order to have adequate time for charting on the computer and sending orders. At present, a computer is the barrier between a doctor and a patient. What we need is to regain the humanity and nobility of this job and maintain our active listening skills. Assigning a scribe for each doctor would definitely help a great deal, in my opinion.

What If Your Days Were Numbered?

"Given enough time, every building collapses, every flower turns to ash, every candle burns out, every name must be forgotten. This is not sad."

- Iain S. Thomas.

The most memorable interaction I had during my clinical rotations was with a patient who was diagnosed with *glioblastoma multiforme*. I went to practice taking history from the ward and was welcomed by the patient's family and the patient himself, a fifty-year-old man lying on the bed, seemingly tired.

Through *history* taking, I discovered that he had had a *stroke* in the past. Only later, while reading his file, did I discover he had that, ironically, terrifying butterfly-shaped glioma. He was one of the 5% of patients who survived this *Malignancy* to live for more than five years. He was back here to be treated for recurrence of the tumour.

What I could not forget was the serene smile he had on his face when I wished him health and recovery. That hope and perseverance taught me what I need to have for my medical career, and that bravery to fight fear every day anchored me on this journey.

The lesson I learned from patients with terminal illnesses: While fighting disease and having a time limit, you can still live the life you've always desired. With their tranquil faces, meaningful gazes, and a hint of a smile, they seem to have a peace of mind that I might have never experienced before.

Compared to them, I feel as though I own everything and have nothing to complain about. And my biggest problems must be so minuscule in comparison. (That oddly gave me relief)

Compared to them, I am guilty of taking my life for granted. Tomorrow is definitely coming. There's no doubt about that. Everything will go as planned. Of course, it will. Except that they have once thought that, too. Until they no longer did.

"An awareness of death encourages us to live more intensely," quoting the Brazilian author Paulo Coelho. I learned through those wonderful people how precious life is and how insignificant it is at the same time. Life is valuable and must be cherished as it is a blessing that is not given to everyone. Every day we breathe is a chance to live our best life. But life is not worth dwelling on. Even while living the brightest moments of our lives, we must not emphasise life. The correct answer, in my opinion, is to detach ourselves from it. To not become enslaved to it, but rather to enjoy it while being aware of its end. Our end.

WHAT CHANGED WASN'T JUST THE MEDICINE

Dr Noor Mohamad Ali

After enduring over one hundred and sixty eight hours of intense pain, worry, confusion, and arguments, a seventy-year-old patient with lower limb *paraesthesia*, *urinary incontinence*, and severe back pain decided to proceed with surgery for her *spinal stenosis* and *disc herniation*. This decision was far from easy due to her existing medical conditions, including *hypertension*, uncontrolled Type II *diabetes*, obesity, and her age, not to mention the risks associated with *anaesthesia* and the surgery itself.

She was placed in a hospital suite where she felt somewhat more comfortable, surrounded by her daughters and granddaughters. Despite the love and support from her family, she felt a deep sense of embarrassment over the need for diaper changes and the *urinary catheter*. Episodes of diarrhoea led to further discomfort as she was unable to clean herself or access the bathroom.

As a medical student, I visited her during morning and evening rounds, as well as for routine check-ups. We've all faced situations where we had to assist elderly family members in challenging circumstances, and it can be uncomfortable. On several occasions, I witnessed her daughter's visible discomfort while changing and cleaning her mother. The patient's own feelings of embarrassment were evident, not to mention the tears that streamed silently down her cheeks.

However, the nurses made a significant difference by asking everyone to step out while they helped the patient change. Their kindness, cheerful demeanour and light-hearted conversation brought a noticeable sense of comfort to the patient.

At that moment, the nurses provided not just medical assistance but also emotional relief, helping her momentarily forget her embarrassment.

While this may not be the most dramatic story, it touched me deeply. It highlighted how simple gestures, comforting words, and a caring attitude can ease a patient's anxiety, especially when facing a major surgery. Bringing joy and comfort to someone undergoing a challenging medical journey is truly a sacred act.

This experience emphasised an essential truth: healthcare providers must do more than diagnose and treat; they must also offer genuine empathy and emotional support. The ability to connect with patients on an emotional level, to provide comfort and dignity in the middle of their struggles, is just as crucial as the clinical care we offer.

Compassionate interactions can profoundly impact a patient's well-being. It is in these moments of vulnerability that our empathy can make the most significant difference, transforming a medical encounter into a deeply supportive experience.

EIGHT MINUTES

Hurairah Faatimah Muzammil

"The highest form of knowledge is empathy, for it requires us to suspend our egos and live in another's world."

- Plato

Oftentimes, as medical students, we are in a flurry to find signs and symptoms, identify sounds, and get to the possible diagnoses, forgetting that they all come from a human. I embodied that mindset - until one *OSCE* station changed everything. We were under tremendous stress, wondering if we could remember the checklists, if we'd get an easy examiner, and so on. On my last station, I went in with the checklist in my mind and ready to "play" the role I needed to for the next eight minutes.

As I introduced myself, took patient demographics, got to the presenting complaint, and reached the middle of my checklist, I realised this was the moment for me to break the bad news to my patient. Something clicked in my head, and I was transported to a hospital where the examiner didn't exist, and the person in front of me was an actual patient.

I distinctly remember that I had to reveal to my patient that she had Stage Four Breast Cancer. In that moment, as the rehearsed words and phrases left my lips, I had the urge to make it right somehow. As I continued recounting the checklist, every action and word felt surreal, as if I were moving through a foggy dream where reality was distant and hazy. My mind raced with thoughts and emotions, struggling to find a balance between my professional facade and the overwhelming sense of responsibility on my shoulders. The sterile environment of the examination room seemed to box me in, amplifying the gravity of the moment, making it feel incredibly intimate and impossibly distant.

As my patient broke down before me, I wanted to rush and give her hope or console her. As she recounted her husband's cancer story and the pain and suffering he went through, I wanted to break down with her; it was as if I could physically feel the pain she was feeling. I could see fear etched into my patient's features, each tear a reminder of her emotional turmoil that accompanies such a devastating diagnosis. I remember dragging my chair closer to her and holding on to her hand. I remember the way she held back tight enough for me to forget that she was playing a role and for me to feel her fear. I can picture my thoughts zeroing in on how broken and afraid she must be, alone, taking in such a grave diagnosis after a traumatic history with her husband. Each time her voice shook as she spoke about her husband with remnants of remembered pain, it became increasingly clear that I wasn't just a doctor who had her clinical duties to perform. I wasn't just a doctor breaking bad news. I was a human being standing before another human being in a moment of profound vulnerability.

But I had a checklist to complete and composure to maintain. As I mechanically went about transitioning into the treatment options, counselling, and referrals, I realised that the patient hadn't left my hand. Her fear was still palpable, her hold unrelenting. In that instant, it hit me - whatever she or I were feeling, my patient would experience tenfold. The more I spoke, the more I realised that no amount of medical jargon or procedural efficiency could truly address the depth of her distress. Her grip was not just symbolic of her fear as she held me as a lifeline; it was a reminder of the trust she placed in me and the immense responsibility I had to carry. While her family and friends would later stand with her, I would be the one she looks to when she's seeking hope and care. It would be me whom she either hopes to meet or dreads to see. The journey ahead for my patient would be fraught with challenges; while I would provide guidance and care, the emotional turmoil she would shoulder would be hers alone. However, it would be up to me to hold her hand through that fear, to guide her to the range of treatment options, support her when things got too hard, and make her as comfortable as I can.

As the bell chimed and the station time was complete, the role player before me snapped out of the scene, while I remained in the previous headspace. The room's atmosphere, previously charged with a whirlwind of emotion, seemed tinged with professional awkwardness. As she released her grip on my hand, I sensed the perceived normality in the environment, while my mind was still reeling. With my emotions running raw, I recollected all those instances in which I had met someone battling cancer. Be it at walks, in the awareness campaigns, or even with my teacher. They projected such a brave mask beyond the pain they held in their hearts. This encounter emphasised the profound responsibility of the role I was to take on, and the depth of connection forged in those fleeting eight minutes. It was the compassionate presence I offered, the empathy I extended, and the human connection I nurtured that would create the true impact of my care. The echoes of her fear and unshed tears in her eyes shall remain with me, a constant reminder of the delicate balance between my professionalism and humanity that defines my life as a doctor.

BEARING WITNESS

Dr Aisha Ismail Makandar

Just like every aspiring medical student/doctor has ever said, 'becoming a doctor was no less than a dream for me.' Even when I started off, I never thought about how much I would earn as a surgeon or how everyone would respect me because I'm a doctor. For me, this noble profession has always been a representation of kindness, care, and dedicated service of the people who are trialled with a prized possession - their health.

Careers in healthcare are widely regarded as some of the most difficult degrees to attain, and I can affirm that from firsthand experience. Underneath all that glamour and academia, people forget about the ruthless journey! Let's put aside the title for a while - my medical journey and the struggles have moulded me into the person I am today. I am honoured to be chosen by Allah for this incredible profession where I can tend to the sick. The countless things that I've not only learned but discovered about myself are way too many to pen down in one excerpt, some of which are still under work with the rigorous cycle of realisation and implementation.

The experiences you go through and the people you meet behind the doors of the hospital become engraved in one's memory for life – you'd be a fool not to take notes!

One such incident fails to leave my memory because of what I could have done if I had recovered from the shock sooner and acted on my initial instinct. I remember that day, that place, that patient, and that expression even to this day. Battling through the traffic, with only coffee to prevent me from dozing off as the car barely moves an inch every few seconds, I arrived at the hospital a few minutes late. We were supposed to be rotating with the *Pulmonology* team that week. That day, the team had a new male patient who had been brought to the hospital from prison as a known case of *Tuberculosis.*

We were instructed by our senior to take a history and examine the patient. He had been kept in an isolation unit and was attached to several monitors, catheters, and a *chest tube* to drain the *hemothorax* (blood in the chest). Dark red blood was trickling down the chest drain into the *underwater seal* container; over 1000 ml of blood had been drained since admission.

We observed all the surroundings with a quick look, noted down our tailored history, and conducted our stepwise physical examination. The patient was unlettered and only spoke in Urdu. It was challenging to explain to him how bad his condition was, especially since he had no family or friends with him at the time. As we were leaving, we called the responsible nurse to ask a few questions. In the meantime, the patient also tried to ask the nurse a few questions, and the next few words that were uttered by the nurse shook me to the core.

"… Anyways, you'll be done for in a few days (an action of slicing his throat) and you'll be packed up in boxes and sent back home on a flight," said the nurse with a small mocking laugh.

I stood there, staring wide-eyed at the nurse's face, and watched him walk away to his workstation to resume work as if this were a daily occurrence for him. I turned to my friend, and we exchanged a look of pure shock mixed with anger and helplessness. We walked away, not knowing how to react, what to say, or how to say it... Can I even say something... Anything?

In today's time, we often love to preach about the glory of justice and the lowliness that lies in injustice. We glorify kindness and look down upon cruelty and misbehaviour. We promote courage and belittle cowardice. We love people who lead with justice and want to punish the oppressors for their wrongdoings. We feed our egos and pride by claiming to be just, kind, and courageous in the face of injustice, cruelty, and oppression. And yet, what about all those moments you just stood by and watched and couldn't say a word? What about the times you hated every second that you witnessed injustice, but couldn't work up the courage to stand up against the oppressor? What about the times you felt powerless in front of someone who was clearly stronger than you? And worst of all, what about the times you chose to stay silent despite all the odds being in your favour? How do you live with that? How does that not shake your conscience every single time your mind thinks of that moment?

Each one of us has witnessed injustice and cruelty around us. Unfortunately, we live in a world where people can say and do bad things. I was then reminded of a *hadith.*

Abu Sa'id reported that The Messenger of Allah, peace and blessings be upon him, said, "Whoever among you sees evil, let him change it with his hand. If he cannot do so, then with his tongue. If he cannot do so, then with his heart, which is the weakest level of faith." (*Ṣaḥīḥ Muslim* 49)

I can never forget or forgive myself, or give a valid excuse for not saying anything in the patient's defence that day. If I ever think of an excuse to justify myself, the only thing I can come up with is, 'I was only a medical student experiencing such an incident for the first time, and I did hate it in my heart.' But that weak excuse always loses its case in the court of my conscience. Nothing justifies treating another human being with cruelty, let alone a sick patient. No degree, no position, no title gives anyone the right to look down upon another human, let alone a patient.

As for us who stand by and watch, please reflect, reflect, and reflect. Would you ever want to be treated that way, and what would you think about the one who stood by and watched? I pray that none of us have a conscience so weak that it doesn't cry in the face of injustice.

A promise to myself: I would NEVER allow myself to stand by and watch someone being treated unjustly or unkindly. I would speak up against the oppressor whenever and wherever needed.

MUSINGS ON THE MOSAIC OF MEDICINE

Dr Mariyam Thahira

When it comes to moments in medicine that left me awestruck, rather than a single grand incident that flashes across the screen of my brain in bold light, I'm overwhelmed by a constellation of experiences and observations that leave me starry-eyed instead. Perhaps, that's how I perceive the field as a whole - a myriad of elements that come together to form a mosaic that's definitely beyond the sum of its parts.

And so, when I ponder upon the factors that accelerated the healing and recovery of the patients that we've seen, I'm humbled by the realisation that many different aspects played a role in paving that path for them. However, what often goes unnoticed are the subtle expressions of compassion from healthcare professionals and the immense comfort they bring to the patients.

One special memory laid the foundation of this principle for me. It was in the *Emergency* department where I was observing surgical *residents* taking care of an elderly woman with an *abscess* (an infected swelling). They were performing a bedside *incision and drainage* procedure, in which a *local anaesthetic* was used before making a small cut over the abscess to release the pus and promote healing. Despite the application of the anaesthetic, certain bedside procedures, such as these, may not be completely pain-free.

Although I've watched procedures like these multiple times in emergency, clouded with the whimpers of the patients and different attempts by the doctors to somewhat console or distract them, this incident was slightly different. Since there were three residents in this particular situation, it was fascinating for me to watch them divide the roles and collaborate. While one of the junior residents took the primary role of doing the procedure and the other junior resident assisted them, the senior resident assumed a dual role, both calmly instructing the junior through the procedure and compassionately offering her hand, providing comfort amidst the pain. The patient grasped the senior resident tightly in order to stay still and to avoid disrupting the procedure. Thanks to their seamless communication and reassuring presence, everything unfolded smoothly.

Once the procedure was over, it was beautiful to see the relief and gratitude of the patient being translated into a string of heartfelt prayers and appreciation. What struck me at that moment was how she thanked the resident who held her hand for emotional support, just as profoundly as she appreciated the resident who performed the procedure.

This left a lasting impression on me as it demonstrated that helping someone heal is often done with the beautiful recipe of combining knowledge and skill, a strong sense of compassion, and a kind way of extending that support to our patients. By doing so, we're reminding them and ourselves, time and time again, that as human beings, we're not just machines which malfunction and require mechanical repair alone. But rather, we're people with minds and souls just as much as physical bodies.

Even when our patients present with physical ailments, we need to imagine, empathise and tend to their psychological and emotional distress as well as give them the space to incorporate their spiritual inclinations. At the end of the day, we're not just here to fix broken parts or glue them together. While that is a service in itself, we should always strive for excellence because, at its core, medicine is not just science but also the delicate art of holding lives together. Perhaps we should take a moment to ensure we allow our patients to heal holistically, knowing all too well that every aspect of their being is interconnected. Once we start doing that, we will begin to realise that the healing this process brings is truly beyond the sum of the efforts we invested!

Certain similar moments along the journey that reinforced this lesson include an encounter in the *labour* room, where I was in awe of my junior, a medical student who would continuously interact with a woman in *labour*, both encouraging her as her spirit began to diminish and explaining to her the importance of certain steps and positions the nurses were encouraging her to try. She was both gentle in her tone and energising in her efforts to motivate, bringing both comfort and clarity to the patient simultaneously.

Another incident occurred just a few floors above, in the *Obstetrics* ward, where a patient with *sickle cell anaemia* was experiencing a *pain crisis* during her pregnancy. In sickle cell *anaemia*, patients may get severe pain in certain parts of the body as the sickle-shaped red blood cells can clog the blood vessels and disrupt blood flow and supply to bones or organs. While she was shivering with pain in a way that even made her jaw rattle, we were awestruck to see her calm down in the moments when a doctor took the time to engage her in a conversation, almost distracting her from the pain altogether!

In a closely related department, the *Neonatal Intensive Care Unit (also called NICU)*, I had the honour of witnessing a moment in slow, cinematic motion that seemed nothing short of magical. There was a beautiful little baby enveloped in the warmth of the *incubator*, who started to get distressed by the *examination* being performed on him by the doctor. However, when the doctor paused his usual steps and just took a moment to place his hand on the baby in an attempt to gently calm him down, I could see his legs, which were floating from the vigorous exertion he had done while crying, slowly fall back down as he became quiet and felt at ease again.

Efforts like these may feel like interruptions to our routine steps, but they're not a hindrance or a burden at all. Rather, they can facilitate our primary objective of restoring our patients' overall health. After all, we've committed ourselves to treading upon this path with the purpose of healing. So, while we're wading along the journey, may we not forget the beautiful intention that we had set out with. May we take the time and effort, invest the thought and emotion to enhance the care we provide by extending our blessed, healing hands, words, tones, expressions, and presence to our patients, thereby relieving their distress and restoring them to full health, or as much of it as we can by God's will.

BEYOND THE STETHOSCOPE

Anonymous

How a Chocolate Bar Solved a Medical Mystery

During my rotation in the *Otorhinolaryngology* (ENT) department, I witnessed a heartwarming incident I'll never forget. A six-year-old girl came to the Outpatient department with her mother, complaining she couldn't eat. Following protocol, the doctor took a detailed history and performed a thorough physical examination to determine the cause.

As I watched, I felt an instant connection with the child. Her presence brightened the clinical atmosphere, and I felt compelled to offer her a chocolate from my pocket. I hesitated, remembering it was *Ramadan*, a month of fasting for Muslims. Yet, an inner voice urged me to make the kind gesture.

To my relief, the girl's mother smiled approvingly when I handed over the chocolate. The child's eyes sparkled as she eagerly unwrapped the treat, savouring each bite with pure delight.

As we watched her enjoy the chocolate, the doctor had a sudden realisation. It became clear that the child's reported inability to eat wasn't due to any medical condition. She simply disliked the food she'd been given at home. This insight brought a collective sense of relief to everyone in the room.

When 'I Am' Becomes 'Am I?' – A Medical Intern's Linguistic Rollercoaster

Being a healthcare provider in the United Arab Emirates requires multilingualism as the country is a melting pot of diverse cultures. I'd like to share a funny incident from one of my training years. Many of my friends speak Malayalam to me, and while I understand the language, I always reply in English.

One day, a patient was admitted to the ICU with *pneumonia.* This patient was articulate and fluent in both Malayalam and English. After the *consultant* doctor and I had taken the important medical *history*, I attempted to introduce myself to the patient in Malayalam, saying, "Nyaan ivda intern aano."

The patient continued the conversation in English, and I realised I'd made a mistake in my sentence. Later, I asked a Malayalam-speaking co-intern how to correctly say "I am an intern here" in Malayalam. They told me it should be "Nyaan ivda internaa."

When I inquired about the difference between "aano" and "aa" at the end of the sentence, the intern explained. How embarrassing! Instead of stating that "I am an intern here," I had inadvertently asked the patient, "Am I an intern here?"

A START, AND MAYBE A CALLING

Dr Mohammed Shaamin

On my first day of internship, I was posted in the *Obstetrics and Gynaecology (OBGYN)* department. To say I was excited would be an understatement. Walking into the ward, I was met with a whirlwind of activity - *residents* and nurses darting up and down, voices overlapping in the chaos of the moment. It was alive, pulsating with energy.

The one who was in charge of orienting us was a second-year resident. She had this unshakeable calm about her, like she's always in control, even when the world is spinning out of order. I'd heard about her before - she once gave *CPR* to her father when he had a *cardiac arrest.* That story stayed with me. Watching her in action today, I could see why people respected her so much. She's one of the best *OBGYN* staff I've met.

As she walked us through the department, I couldn't help but wonder how much I'd be able to contribute as a male *intern* in this specialty. Would the patients trust me? Would they be comfortable with me around? These questions lingered at the back of my mind, but I tried to focus on the task at hand, soaking in every detail of the orientation.

About half an hour into my first shift, I heard the nurse calling me frantically. She asked me to come take a look at one of the patients. I nodded, masking my nervousness with what I hoped was a calm appearance.

"What happened?" I asked as she guided me to the patient. The woman before me was fully pregnant, crying out in pain. My heart raced. "What's wrong?" I asked, my voice sounding steadier than I actually felt. The nurse pulled back the blankets, and I froze for a split second. The baby's head was already *crowning*.

"Let's move!" someone shouted, and everything became a blur. We rushed her to the *labour room*. My mind was racing, but my hands moved instinctively, following the team's lead. The delivery was surprisingly smooth – quick, calm, almost effortless in the end.

As I stood there later, watching the new life take its initial breaths, I felt something stir deep within me. Love, respect, a strange sense of belonging. In that moment, I felt connected to the department, to the team, to the work itself.

Fast forward to now. I've completed my internship, and *OBGYN* is still my favourite department from the *internship*, and that *resident* is still my most beloved mentor. Maybe, just maybe, this could be my specialty. Who knows?

REKINDLING EMPATHY IN A DISCONNECTED WORLD

Sobia Mir

My desire to pursue medicine stems from a journey of self-discovery that transformed my perception of sensitivity and empathy. As a child, my emotional nature often made me feel out of place in a world that seemed to value stoicism over compassion. However, a pivotal experience during a visit to Kashmir when I was twelve years old changed everything. My family is from Kashmir, and we were visiting relatives when I accompanied my grandfather to a hospital to get medication for his eyes.

Upon entering the hospital, I was struck by the overwhelming atmosphere of fatigue and despair. Long queues of tired patients filled the hallways, many of whom had travelled from rural areas in hopes of receiving medical care. The air was heavy with a sense of urgency as individuals awaited their turn, their faces a mix of anxiety and weariness. As I observed this scene, I began to notice the doctors moving quickly through their consultations, their faces etched with the strain of overwork and frustration. It felt as though they were simply going through the motions, prescribing medications in haste without truly connecting with the people before them. Watching this unfold, I couldn't help but wonder if the doctors even cared about what they were prescribing. I felt a deep sense of disconnection between the doctors and the patients; between the act of healing and the human touch it requires.

At the time, I didn't fully understand the reasons behind this rushed, impersonal care. But as I've grown older and more aware of the world, I've come to realise that this overmedicalisation was a product of systemic inefficiencies in the healthcare system. The hospital experience served as a stark reminder of how deeply interconnected healthcare is with societal factors, and I began to see the significance of empathy in this context.

Kashmir's healthcare system is plagued by various challenges, with a doctor-patient ratio far below the World Health Organisation's recommendations. This scarcity leads to significant strain on medical professionals, who find themselves overwhelmed with patients. Many doctors prioritise private practice, resulting in government hospitals being understaffed and under-resourced. Consequently, patients who rely on public healthcare often find themselves at a disadvantage, facing long waiting times and a lack of personalised care.

The environment I witnessed was a microcosm of these larger systemic issues. The long lines and hurried consultations reflected not just a lack of resources but also an urgent need for a more compassionate approach to medicine. Patients were treated as numbers rather than individuals, their unique stories overlooked in the rush to prescribe medications. This overmedicalisation can lead to a cycle where patients feel dissatisfied with their care, which can further exacerbate their health issues.

What struck me most during my visit was not just the inefficiency of the healthcare system, but the emotional toll it took on both patients and providers. The hurried consultations I observed highlighted how overburdened healthcare systems often neglect the emotional and psychological needs of patients. It became clear to me that many of the individuals in the waiting room were not just suffering from physical ailments; they were grappling with the weight of their circumstances, both in terms of health and the societal conditions surrounding them.

This realisation prompted me to reflect on my own experiences. My sensitivity, which I once perceived as a weakness, began to emerge as a source of strength. Until then, I had always been told that being too emotional would hold me back, especially in a field like medicine. However, witnessing the disconnection between doctors and patients in that hospital made me realise that empathy - the very thing I had been told was a liability - was, in fact, a powerful tool for healing. I understood that in a world that often capitalises on disconnection, cultivating empathetic connections is paramount. My sensitivity allowed me to connect with the patients' unspoken emotions, recognising their pain and frustration in ways that went beyond mere physical symptoms.

This experience fundamentally shaped the way I approach my medical education. I no longer see medicine as simply a science of diagnosing and treating diseases; I see it as an opportunity to bridge the gap between patient and practitioner. I believe that true healing requires a holistic approach, one that treats not just the illness, but the person behind it.

I aspire to foster a healthcare environment where empathy is prioritised, and patients are viewed as partners in their own care. It is crucial for healthcare providers to invest time in understanding the stories of their patients, creating a space where individuals feel valued and heard. Through my journey in medicine, I aim to advocate for patient-centred care, focusing not just on curing disease but on healing the whole person - emotionally, physically, and mentally.

As I continue my medical education, I am inspired by the belief that sensitivity and emotional intelligence are invaluable tools in fostering genuine healing. I strive to create an atmosphere where patients feel empowered, knowing that their concerns are acknowledged and addressed. It is imperative that we move away from a model of care that emphasises efficiency and speed, towards one that values connection and understanding.

In a world that often prioritises efficiency over connection, I am committed to being a force for change in the healthcare landscape. My experience in Kashmir has instilled in me a deep desire to ensure that the next generation of healthcare providers understands that healing is not just about treating the body – it's about touching the heart. By cultivating empathy in medical practice, we can create a more compassionate healthcare system that recognises the humanity of every patient.

Ultimately, I aim to be the kind of doctor who not only treats illness but also nurtures the emotional well-being of my patients. I envision a future where healthcare is not merely transactional, but relational - a space where empathy thrives, and healing is holistic. My journey in medicine is just beginning, and I carry with me the lessons learned from that hospital visit, determined to make a difference in the lives of those I serve.

THE CHILD WITHIN

Dr Ahila Abu-Nayla

In the demanding world of medical training, the focus often lies on attaining knowledge, honing clinical skills, and the endless pursuit of academic excellence. As medical students, we are advised to invest our time in religiously studying and striving for perfection in our future careers as physicians. However, amidst the chaos of our desire for academic recognition, we overlook moments that highlight the true essence of medicine - the moments that can't be found in the confines of textbooks or lecture halls.

This essay illustrates a personal encounter with a five-year-old *leukaemia* fighter whose bright spirit and touching words left an indelible mark on my approach to medical care. It was a mundane day in the *Paediatric Oncology* ward, a place where the fragility of life is juxtaposed with the resilience of the human spirit. My day was filled with the usual ward round, case discussions, and the reminder of an upcoming lecture at the back of my head. I was particularly looking forward to the lecture that afternoon as it was a crucial topic for my approaching exams. However, fate had different plans for me. It intended to teach me a valuable lesson that day.

As I moved through the ward, checking on patients and revising notes, I noticed a little girl sitting in her bed, her head bowed as she concentrated on a colouring book. Her name was Sarah, and at five years old, she was in the middle of a battle with cancer – a battle that had stolen her hair, her energy, and confined her to a hospital bed. Yet, as I got closer to her, I was surprised by her bright attitude.

I greeted her and introduced myself as a medical student to Sarah. She looked up at me with a warm smile, full of curiosity, showing no hint of the usual reluctance displayed by other children in the hospital. It was apparent to me that, despite her physical condition, her spirit was still as vibrant as ever.

Our conversation soon turned to the future, and I asked Sarah what she wanted to be when she grew up. Without hesitation, she replied, "I want to be a nurse." Her answer took me by surprise. Curious, I asked her why she didn't want to be a doctor instead, after all, she was speaking to an aspiring physician. After a thoughtful pause, she replied with a clarity that struck me deeply, "Because nurses care more about me. The doctors don't."

Her words were simple, yet they carried a heavy message. In that moment, Sarah reminded me of a crucial part of patient care that's often overlooked in the world of medicine, buried among the toils of challenging exams and long work hours. With all her innocence, she highlighted to me the importance of dedicating time, attention, and the human connection in our daily practice. She expressed dejection about how doctors seemed to care more about the numbers rather than talking to her and claimed they spent more time talking to her mother rather than communicating with her. As she spoke, I could feel the weight of her words settling over me, and I realised that there was more to this encounter than a simple conversation.

As Sarah and I continued to talk, I felt a growing sense of uneasiness within me. On one hand, I knew I had a lecture to attend, one that was important for my academic progress. The rational part in me urged me to stick to my schedule and to leave the ward in time for my lecture. On the other hand, I was disappointed that a little girl yearned for attention, for someone to spend time with her, and to make her feel seen and valued. Her words about only nurses seeming to care about her echoed in my mind. I couldn't shake the feeling that I would be letting her down like all the others had and that leaving her now would be a missed opportunity, not just for her, but for me as well.

After an internal struggle, I made my decision. I pulled up a chair and asked if I could join her in colouring. Her face lit up in a smile that instantly washed away all the doubts I had about missing the lecture. She handed me a crayon, and together we began to colour, filling the pages with vibrant hues. Colouring with Sarah was more than just filling the pages of a book - it was as if she was colouring my life, adding vibrant hues to my perspective and making me appreciate the smaller things. Each stroke of her crayons and each heartfelt laugh coming from her reminded me of the simple joys and the profound impact of taking the time to connect with others, even in the midst of life's challenges.

As we coloured, our conversations flowed naturally. Sarah told me more about her dream of becoming a nurse, expressing her admiration for their work ethic and how they cared for her, always making time to listen, comfort, and be there when she needed them. I realised how doctors, with their often-hurried schedules, sometimes overlook the importance of personal touch and forget the significance of forming a connection with their patients.

We also raced down the corridor of the ward, our laughter echoing through the sterile hallways. In that brief moment, I allowed myself to become a child alongside Sarah, shedding the weight of my lab coat and all the responsibilities it represents. It was a fleeting, playful escape that reminded me of the importance of living fully in the moment, especially when that moment brings a smile to a child's face.

During our brief encounter, I realised that healing is not restricted to the administration of treatments or the performance of procedures. Healing in its truest sense is about addressing the whole person – their physical, emotional, and psychological needs. In addition, it is about being present, listening, and offering comfort to patients and their families in their time of need.

Eventually, the time came for me to leave. I had spent far longer with Sarah than I had originally planned, and I knew that I had missed the lecture. But as I said goodbye and promised to visit her again, I felt no regret. Instead, I felt a deep sense of fulfilment, knowing that I made the right choice not just for Sarah, but for myself as well. As I was leaving the ward, Sarah smiled and said, "Maybe not all doctors are the same. Some of them do care." Her words were the perfect reminder that the connections we make can change perceptions and, more importantly, bring comfort and trust to those who need it the most.

As I walked out of the ward, I reflected on the experience and the lessons I had learned. Missing the lecture, in the grand scheme of things, seemed unimportant compared to the opportunity I had been given to connect with Sarah. This experience underlined a fundamental truth about healthcare: the importance of compassionate care. In the fast-paced world of modern medicine focused on efficacy and outcomes, we often forget the importance of human connection and empathy. We fail to acknowledge the unique needs of each patient and understand that patients are not mere cases or conditions but individuals with hopes, fears, and dreams, just like Sarah, yearning to be seen, heard, and valued.

As I continue my journey to Medicine, I carry with me the lessons I learned from Sarah. I am more conscious of my attitude and more mindful of taking the time to connect with patients. In the end, the true measure of success in medicine is not just the number of lectures attended or grades achieved, but the lives we touch, the comfort we provide, and the humanity we bring to practice. I owe my knowledge of this truth to a little girl fighting her own battles, steadfast despite her frail body, and to her, I am eternally grateful.

A HOLISTIC PERSPECTIVE

Dr Tasnim Mustafa and Rushda Haider

When we hear the word "doctor," what comes to your mind?

Well, some may describe the doctor as a person who treats people. However, in my understanding, being a doctor is much more than that. They are highly trained medical professionals who diagnose illnesses, provide treatments, offer preventive care, and support patients' overall well-being. In addition to their medical expertise, showing empathy is a fundamental aspect of being a doctor. Empathy allows doctors to understand and connect with their patients on an emotional level, fostering trust and improving patient care. By demonstrating empathy, doctors can better appreciate their patients' concerns, fears, and experiences, which enhances communication and ensures that patients feel heard and valued. This compassionate approach is essential for providing holistic care that addresses not only the physical but also the emotional and psychological needs of the patients.

The way doctors approach their patients is crucial, as it significantly impacts the diagnosis process. When doctors show empathy and are attentive listeners, patients are more likely to open up and provide detailed information about their symptoms and experiences. This open communication helps doctors gather the necessary details to accurately diagnose the illness. Therefore, being a doctor involves a combination of medical knowledge, empathy, communication skills, and a commitment to lifelong learning and patient advocacy.

As a medical student, I have personally observed the vital role empathy plays in diagnosing illnesses and achieving positive outcomes. During my time in the hospital, I observed a patient who initially provided the doctor with a brief summary of his complaint. The doctor approached him with empathy, which made the patient feel more comfortable. As a result, the patient shared more detailed information, which ultimately helped the doctor analyse the situation thoroughly and provide the best treatment. Another patient came in for her first delivery, and the entire team was incredibly empathetic and supportive. Their care made her feel stronger and happier, allowing her to navigate the unforgettable journey of childbirth with greater ease.

From a patient's perspective, my experience during my *tonsillectomy* highlighted the impact of empathy. I was filled with anxiety and fear, but the nurse and doctor continuously checked on me and reassured me throughout the process. Their care transformed my journey from one of fear to one of gratitude and thankfulness, making me realise the profound impact of empathy.

This demonstrates that communication skills, being good listeners, and empathy play crucial parts in our roles as medical professionals. Our healing hands are not just for administering treatment, but also for nurturing and healing the soul. Furthermore, in today's high-tech medical world, it is easy to overlook the importance of human connection. However, I have repeatedly witnessed how kindness, family support, empathy, and a personal touch can significantly impact healing.

One of my most memorable experiences involved an elderly patient who felt lonely and anxious. After a tough day, I took a moment to hold her hand and listen. To me, it was a small act of kindness, but to her, it was a lifeline. She later shared how that simple gesture made her feel truly cared for. It reminded me that a little kindness can be as powerful as any medication. Family support is another critical piece of the healing puzzle. The love and presence of family can create a nurturing environment that accelerates recovery. Their presence and encouragement give strength and hope, proving that healing is not just physical but deeply emotional as well.

Humanising medicine is equally important. While technology plays a crucial role in diagnosing and treating patients, it lacks the warmth and understanding needed for true healing. I remember a young mother with her sick child, overwhelmed by the medical jargon and machines. Taking the time to explain things in simple terms and offer emotional support helped bridge the gap between technology and the human touch. This taught me that while technology is essential, it is the personal connection and empathy that truly make medicine work.

Achieving compassionate medicine while respecting differences in the population is important. Cultural sensitivity in patient care is essential for providing effective and compassionate treatment. It involves recognising and respecting the diverse cultural backgrounds, beliefs, and practices of patients. This awareness allows healthcare professionals to tailor their care to meet the unique needs and preferences of each individual.

Empathy is closely linked to cultural sensitivity. By showing empathy, healthcare providers can better understand and appreciate the cultural contexts that shape their patients' experiences, values, and expectations. This understanding fosters a stronger patient-doctor relationship, as patients feel seen, heard, and respected. For example, certain cultural beliefs may influence how patients perceive illness, pain, or medical interventions. An empathetic and culturally sensitive healthcare provider will take the time to listen to these concerns and incorporate them into the treatment plan. This approach not only enhances patient satisfaction but also improves adherence to medical advice and outcomes.

Moreover, cultural sensitivity helps prevent misunderstandings and potential biases that could negatively impact patient care. It encourages open communication, reduces health disparities, and promotes a more inclusive and supportive healthcare environment. In summary, cultural sensitivity and empathy are intertwined in patient care. Together, they enable healthcare professionals to deliver personalised, respectful, and effective treatment, ultimately leading to better patient experiences and health outcomes.

Compassion can also serve as a powerful tool in overcoming burnout. Addressing burnout, characterised by emotional exhaustion, depersonalisation, and a diminished sense of personal accomplishment, is increasingly important in the medical field due to its prevalence among healthcare professionals. Integrating compassion into their practice can effectively counteract burnout's detrimental effects. Compassion for patients involves understanding their suffering, being present, and taking action to alleviate it. When healthcare providers practice compassion, they often find their work more meaningful, which can regenerate their sense of purpose and dedication, thereby relieving and lessening burnout.

Self-compassion is equally vital. Healthcare professionals often hold themselves to high standards and may neglect their own well-being. By practising self-compassion, they can acknowledge their challenges and treat themselves with the same kindness they offer their patients. This involves recognising the importance of self-care, setting healthy boundaries, and seeking support when needed. Team compassion also plays a crucial role. A supportive work environment where colleagues show empathy and understanding toward each other can help alleviate the stress and isolation that contribute to burnout. Encouraging open communication, mutual support, and shared responsibility fosters a collaborative atmosphere that significantly reduces burnout rates.

Incorporating mindfulness and stress-reduction techniques into daily routines can further enhance compassionate care. Practices such as meditation, deep breathing, and reflective journaling help healthcare providers stay centred and resilient, allowing them to approach their work with renewed energy and empathy. Compassion not only enhances patient care but also serves as a potent antidote to burnout among healthcare professionals. By prioritising compassion for patients, practising self-compassion, fostering a supportive team environment, and embracing mindfulness, healthcare providers can effectively combat burnout and sustain their well-being in demanding clinical settings.

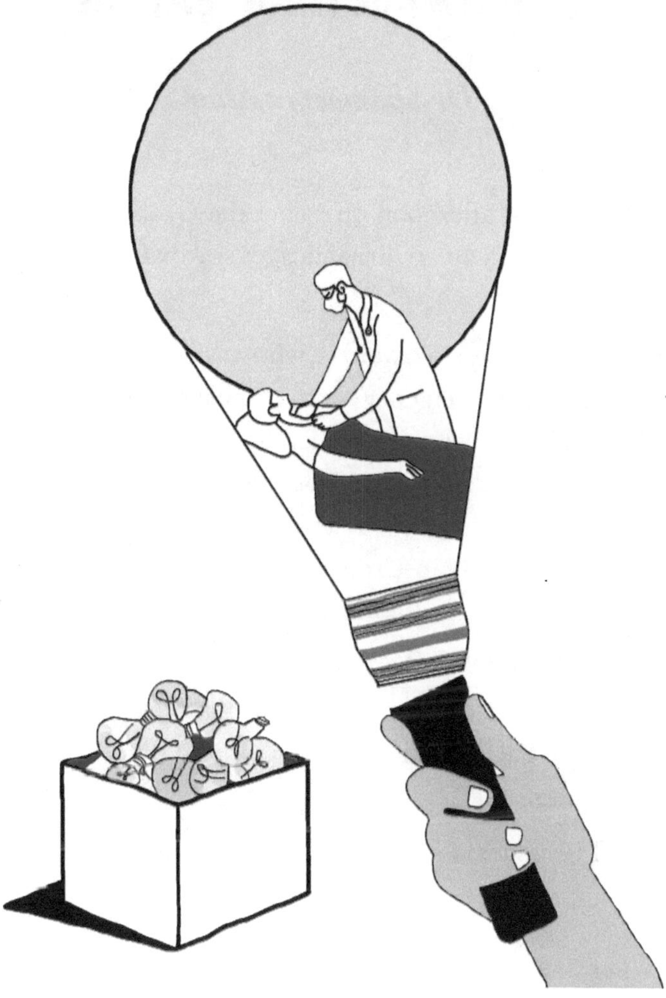

LOSS AND THE LIGHT LEFT BEHIND

EMPATHY IN TRANSLATION

Dr Shameema Alam

I attended my last afternoon on-call at the *Gynaecology* emergency in a hospital. It was a very dynamic, yet sorrowful experience for me.

A twenty-four-year-old woman, who was eleven weeks pregnant, was brought to the emergency room complaining of constant left-sided lower abdominal pain, tenderness, vomiting, and shoulder pain. She and her relatives were not able to speak in English; they only spoke Urdu. Since no one else could communicate with the patient and her family in Urdu, I stepped in as an interpreter. I translated her words to the doctor and reassured her when her voice quivered with uncertainty.

The ultrasound confirmed what we had feared - a ruptured *ectopic pregnancy*. She needed immediate surgery. But before that, she needed answers.

"Will I be under *anaesthesia*?" she whispered.

"Will it hurt?"

"Will I survive? Will I go back home to my little daughter?"

I hesitated for a fraction of a second, then looked into her tear-filled eyes and tried my best to comfort her.

Her family was just as desperate for answers. Would she make it? Would she ever conceive again? I relayed their concerns to the doctors and their reassurances back to them. In that moment, I wasn't just a medical student - I was their only connection to hope.

After the successful completion of the surgery, I was given the task of conveying the findings of the operation and the result to the patient's family, who were waiting outside the operating theatre. I showed them all the photographs from the operation to describe what occurred to the patient during that procedure inside the theatre. I also clarified any questions they had.

Overall, the patient's condition was heartbreaking. I was unhappy and pitiful to see her in such agony. I felt dejected because, just as she was celebrating the good news of becoming a mother, an ectopic pregnancy turned her world upside down, necessitating the removal of her fallopian tube in order to save her health.

Even though I'll never truly understand how she must be feeling, I was able to empathise with her and console her before the operation. Furthermore, I was eager to witness my first *gynaecological laparoscopic* surgery. This incident not only allowed me to see a real-life management of an ectopic pregnancy but also a chance to contribute to taking history from the patient, conveying and explaining critical information, gaining consent for surgery, and counselling the family after the surgery.

That day, I witnessed both the fragility of life and the power of human connection. Medicine isn't just about knowledge or technical skills – it's about presence. In a moment of crisis, I wasn't the most senior person in the room, and yet, I was the one who could bring comfort and clarity to a frightened mother and her family.

FINDING LIGHT IN THE DARKNESS

Dr Salam C. Kandi

It was a weekend past midnight, in the doctors' *ER* duty room of a hospital in a coastal city of India, when I, a *resident* at that time, received the call to procure eyes from a deceased lady. I travelled by the hospital vehicle to the suburbs. Heavy rain poured relentlessly, as if washing away the grime of the city streets. I hurried through the downpour. My umbrella could barely hold up against the gusts of wind.

As I arrived at the small, weathered house, I was greeted by the woman's son, Rahul, who led me inside. The interior was cosy, with the scent of frankincense mingling with the dampness brought in from outside. I set up my equipment with care, while the dim light from a nearby lamp cast long shadows on the walls.

The deceased woman lay peacefully, her face serene despite the storm raging outside. Her eyes were closed, and her hands folded gently over her chest. Rahul stood silently beside her, his expression a mix of sorrow and gratitude. "Thank you for coming, Dr Salam," Rahul whispered. "My mother wanted to give the gift of sight even in passing." I nodded solemnly, feeling the weight of the responsibility. As I prepared for the procedure, I focused on the task ahead, knowing the profound impact this donation would have on others.

The procedure began, and each step was meticulous and deliberate. The quietness of the house was punctuated only by the occasional patter of raindrops against the windowpanes. With utmost care, I performed the delicate process of removing the eyes, knowing these precious gifts would soon bring light to two young patients who desperately needed them.

As I placed the eyes gently in the preservation solution, I felt a sense of reverence for the woman's final act of kindness. Her selfless donation would restore vision to others, enabling them to see the world anew. Having completed the procedure, I stepped back, my heart heavy with the solemnity of the moment. Rahul stood by his mother's bedside, with his eyes moist with tears. He said softly, "My mother's gift will change lives."

Leaving the small house, the rain had begun to subside, leaving behind a quiet calmness. I stood on the doorstep, watching as the clouds parted to reveal a patch of dawn. In that moment, I felt a deep sense of gratitude, not just for the opportunity to honour this woman's wish, but for the profound reminder of the power of generosity and compassion.

The donated eyes would soon find new homes, bringing clarity and colour to lives that had only known darkness. And I, with each step I took in my journey as a doctor, would carry the memory of this day, the day I was entrusted with a gift that transcended life and death, given by a woman who had left a legacy of kindness and hope.

SCREAMS AND WAILS

Dr Aya Mohammed Ali Alsabbah

"A wonderful fact to reflect upon is that every human creature is constituted to be that profound secret and mystery to every other"

– Charles Dickens

However, as physicians, we get to be part of their story briefly, either at its darkest or brightest. One day at work is enough to not only witness death and sorrow but also embrace new lives and joy. Time conducts its magic and creates indifference in the heart, as repeated exposure to such events leads to desensitisation - where barely any compassion is felt for others' misery, and barely any joy resonates with others' happiness. Most healthcare providers work with such emptiness within until, occasionally, an incident like no other delves deep into their hearts, evoking dormant emotions.

The heroine of one such incident was a brave young mother who was still oblivious to the cruelty of reality. The circumstance in which I met her was quite unusual. In fact, our acquaintance must have been during the worst hours of her life, or so it seemed.

At the time when I was still a medical student in my final years, the gleaming summer sun was approaching as June had begun. I had already been stationed in the *Obstetrics and Gynaecology* (OBGYN) department for two months, where all was going smoothly until the afternoon of a certain Monday.

On that day, I had checked the patients before the *rounds*, participated actively during the rounds, and then accompanied the residents as they were documenting. We were leisurely discussing the types of miscarriage until dreadful screams filled the Obstetrics ward, where shouting, screaming, and yelling were regular sounds. However, these ghastly screams were different. Devastation and desperation filled the air as nurses pushed the bed of a woman towards the ICU. No features of the woman were visible from the long, dim hairs covering her face as she howled and wailed in horror, desperately wrapping her arms around what seemed to be a towel on her chest.

My colleague, Sara, and I had taken a few steps back from the intensity of the scene and the loud screams because of which we had to cover our ears. Although what happened occurred in a few seconds, it had felt like three hours, if not more.

Sara: *What exactly happened?*

Me: *Absolutely no clue. Whatever it is, I'm sure it's horrendous.*

As we were approaching the end of the day, we each went home preoccupied with thoughts about this poor woman, oblivious of what had occurred to her until the next day.

On Tuesday, the same routine resumed, with the priority being the admitted patients. Sara and I postponed all the questions and uncertainties held from the day before until proper care was delivered to the patients we had been assigned for the day. After rounds, we finally had the opportunity to ask the consultant about the peculiar incident.

Consultant: *Alright, I'll tell you what happened so that you'll be aware of such cases if you meet any in the future. But let's head to a room since such confidential matters can't be discussed in the corridor for the patient's autonomy and privacy.*

Let us call our patient Lily. She is a previously healthy twenty-year-old who was a victim of child marriage. Forced to marry at fifteen years old against her will, her life with her husband wasn't as bad as she had imagined. But that soon changed when a whole year had passed without any announcement of pregnancy, and her in-laws demanded to marry their son to a second wife to bear his offspring. Other major obstacles and problems intervened with the married couple's life until, after five long years, the most awaited news reached her parents and in-laws - she was finally bearing a child.

Me: *Then, isn't that some happy news? Why was she in that condition? Did something happen?*

Consultant: *Well, there is still a lot to be told...*

Once the elders in the couple's family knew about the pregnancy, they decided to move in with them to take care of Lily. Unfortunately, the confirmation of pregnancy was only through a regular test, and from that day until today, she hasn't seen a doctor. No prenatal care, no ultrasound, and no basic investigations were done until she felt contractions. After nine months, Lily went into labour, but it seemed prolonged, which worried the family members, causing them to bring her to our hospital.

Sara: *Is the baby alive? Please don't say otherwise.*

Consultant: *He is... at least, currently.*

Me: *Why does that seem ominous, Doctor? Isn't he fine?*

Consultant: *I told you that it's a long story. When Lily arrived at our emergency room, we quickly evaluated her condition. Her blood pressure was very high. My team and I suspected Pre-eclampsia. A third-year resident was performing the ultrasound at that time to check the baby. She took an awfully long time staring at the screen until I reminded her of the urgency of the situation. That's when she turned around with an aghast face.*

Resident: *Oh, Doctor, please take a look…*

Consultant: *Once I saw the screen, I knew exactly why her face was colourless. But before I could say anything, Lily's heartbeats began decreasing, and we had to rush her to the operating room.*

Anencephaly…

A baby boy was safely delivered; he had two eyes, a nose, a mouth, and two sets of ears, but no skull. He was not breathing, so he was directly shifted to the neonatal ICU. With the necessary interventions, he became stable. The mother could not see her son until she was shifted to the obstetric ward, which was a few minutes before you saw her. Unaware of his condition and after a tough pregnancy journey, Lily couldn't tolerate the news. Thus was her reaction that you saw…"

A moment of silence went by while Sara and I were trying to comprehend what the doctor was saying.

Sara: *Doctor, how is he alive if he doesn't have a brain? Can he live long?*

I nodded along while Sara was asking, since the same questions crossed my mind.

Consultant: *The main systems that keep the body alive are controlled by the brain stem, which the baby does have. However, it is expected that he would pass away anytime from now in the coming few days."*

We parted from the doctor as she had an emergency case to tend to, still in shock from what we had heard. Pity, sadness, and dejection filled us as we made our way to the cafeteria, silently pondering how crestfallen Lily must be while waiting for her son's inevitable death. The loss of a son and the confronting, judging eyes of the family elders were things that she had to face.

When I pondered this encounter later on, however, I also realised the importance of *antenatal care*, early diagnosis, and the necessary skill of breaking bad news to patients and their families.

Although some consider ignorance to be a blessing, it may not always be true. A mother usually forms a deep connection with the baby in her womb before birth, thus harbouring immense affection. When combined with the anticipation for the baby's arrival, this creates great fears for the new mother regarding any minute issue during her pregnancy.

Preparing a person like that, who may be brimming with excitement and anxiety alike, to receive the most tragic news of their life is one of the fundamental practices that a doctor must perfect, and students should be taught early. Moreover, providing appropriate care and regular check-ups before pregnancy would have been monumental in allowing the mother to feel emotionally prepared and socially supported, even if the medical outcome remains unchanged.

Early diagnosis, hand in hand with delivering the news professionally, and additional family counselling would indeed improve the patient's emotional outcome and soften their reception of such devastating news.

HOW BUGSY GOT ITS NAME

Dr Shyam Kishan

Years ago, I was working as a Spine Surgeon at a bustling academic Children's Hospital. One day, I picked up the intake form for a new patient, a fifteen-year-old girl, and noticed that her *chief complaint* was listed as "I am dying!" followed by a slew of exclamation marks. Teenagers can be dramatic, often declaring they're "dying" over something minor, so I didn't give it much thought.

When I entered her room, I found it shrouded in darkness, with the curtains drawn tight. There was a small figure lying on the examination table, bundled up in a blanket. I gently woke her, revealing a frail girl who looked younger than her listed fifteen years. She was bald, clearly from *chemotherapy*.

She sat up, and after I introduced myself, I asked why she was there to see me. With a calmness that took me by surprise, she explained that someone thought I should see her because her recurrent *mediastinal rhabdomyosarcoma* (muscular tumour) was pressing against her spine. The truth of her *chief complaint* hit me hard - she really was dying.

I spent almost an hour talking with her and her mother, and somewhere in that conversation, she decided I was worth talking to. She was so full of life, so spirited, that I couldn't help but comment on her incredible vitality. She shot back, "Duh! If I weren't so full of life, I'd already be dead."

At one point, she looked at me and asked, "Do you have a name for that thing?" I was confused, so I asked what she meant. She pointed at my moustache and said, "That thing on your upper lip." I told her I hadn't thought about naming my moustache before. She studied it for a moment and then declared, "It looks like a Bugsy." And just like that, my moustache had a name.

A few weeks later, she passed away. I still treasure the brief time I had with her. She taught me so much about grace, peace, and dignity, about accepting life and death with a wisdom far beyond her years. She wasn't afraid, just tired, yet still so joyful.

I think of her every now and then, the girl who named my moustache.

READ AT YOUR OWN RISK

Dr Shaista Khadim

Everyone has their firsts; for medical students, the firsts are usually different, difficult, scary, and unexpected. From the first time seeing a *cadaver* to the first time witnessing death, these firsts are not fun to remember. But we don't forget them either. Never.

The first time we stood in front of a cadaver and were introduced to the name and mode of death of the body in front of us, we felt squirmy from within. Even the humorous ones in our group were dead serious. At least we were together, in a group, with our friends while witnessing this first - that was the only comfort.

But when you witness your first death, you are alone.

It doesn't matter how many people you are surrounded by when it happens; suddenly, it's just you, your patient who just breathed their last, and the Angel of Death in that space.

Back in my fourth year of medical school, I had done an elective rotation in the *Internal Medicine* department where I was assigned to be in *Emergency* one day. A fifteen-year-old girl was rushed into Emergency that day, accompanied by her father and *paramedics* from the ambulance. She was unconscious and had a very high body temperature.

Initial history revealed that she was a patient of *AML (Acute Myeloid Leukaemia)*: a type of blood cancer of the white blood cells, and was on *chemotherapy*. She was *vitally unstable* and unresponsive to our calls. We diagnosed her with *febrile neutropenia* (fever in people who have low neutrophil count due to chemotherapy) based on initial labs. This is an *oncological* emergency and should be dealt with immediately. We started her on antibiotics and other supportive management. But she soon crashed, and *code blue* was announced.

I was assigned to a different bed, so I stayed there and observed it all from a distance. I'll be honest, I was scared to go closer. I watched as the team of doctors rushed to start CPR *(cardiopulmonary resuscitation)* on the patient. The father stood by the foot of the bed, constantly muttering something under his breath, hands shaking, eyes watering, and face looking more ashen than his daughter's.

As the doctors took turns doing the CPR, my senior caught my eye and beckoned me to join the team. I shook my head, and he continued with the CPR. A few moments later, he looked at me again, and this time, he gave me a stern look. And so, I budged.

I took quick steps and reached the bed. I stood opposite my senior. He finished his round and beckoned me to start, and I did. After one round of CPR, I changed places with another doctor. The CPR went on for what seemed like aeons. There was no change in her clinical condition; her heartbeat didn't return, and her chest never rose. The final checking of *brainstem reflexes* revealed that she was no more.

I got out of the crowd and tried to find a chair because my legs felt like jelly. I had never known what taking heavy steps meant. Never knew what stalling of time felt like. Never knew what frozen surroundings looked like until then. The room seemed to close upon me. I needed to leave and find some air. So, instead of sitting, I kept walking, out of Emergency into the sun. I felt my eyes stinging - sun or tears - I didn't know. I stood there as the world continued at its pace around me.

Soon, I made my way back to the Emergency. She lay there, peacefully. (My hands shake as I write this now.) Her father sat beside her, tears streaming down his face as he stared at his daughter. He slowly got up, touched her face gently, and then covered it.

No one can get close to what would be going on in the mind of the father who just lost his lovely daughter. Did his world come crashing down on him? Did he secretly thank God she was free of all pain? What was he thinking? Why was his face so calm?

As doctors, we learn from every patient who comes to us, just so we can do better when a similar patient comes to us in the future. But what is there to learn from a patient we lost? In a patient, we tried to do our best to save? We learn that life can be brutal. But it is also beautiful.

THROUGH THE CRACK IN THE BLUE DOORS

Dr Rawan Ahmed Mehanna

Medical *Intern* Officer Logs: *ER* Department, Night Shift - 10:00 p.m.

For Non-Medics, this may sound horrific, but for those of us in the *ER*, this is, unfortunately, a normal occurrence. I loved working night shifts long before I even experienced them. *ER* Resus night shifts, in particular, always held a special place in my heart. On some nights, you come across two to three patients throughout your entire shift, while on other nights, like the one I'm about to recount, you see a myriad of cases unfolding simultaneously.

As I was casually finishing up suturing a head wound in Room One, the shift captain instructed me to go observe the case of *supraventricular tachycardia (SVT)* that had just arrived in the other room. This is not uncommon in such shifts; the arrival of patients can overlap with one another. Turning my attention to Room Two, I joined my *attending* to the case and started my assessment of the patient's history and examination.

Engrossed as we were, there was a sudden swoosh of the resus doors, and the mad scramble of frantic footsteps was inescapable. A *gurney* was pushed into Room One, heading straight for bed 1A. Family members and the other night shift team crowded around the bed.

It was a *cardiac arrest.*

In that instant, my body was flooded with an overwhelming mix of adrenaline, apprehension, and dread. This is a moment every *intern* prepares for and thinks about but can never truly be ready to face. I remember my mentor gave me a quick look with her face fixed on the patient; it was obvious those eyes had years of experience that could bring something I could only aspire to achieve.

Since another doctor was handling the cardiac arrest, we stayed with our patient battling the supraventricular tachycardia. Thankfully, our patient was stabilised and the adrenaline was beginning to wind down. Yet, I remember how I felt suspended between two worlds: the controlled chaos of managing SVT with my mentor and the impending storm that was about to crash into the opposite room. Knowing that in one room we were pulling someone back from the brink of death and in another, someone was teetering on the edge, unknown, unseen.

I can't even remember exactly how long it was from the moment we got the call to the moment I saw the patient being pushed through the doors - time in the ER seems to both stretch and compress all at once. I glanced through the narrow opening of the door in that room (after the team ordered it closed) and saw the patient. He was motionless and looked like he was simply sleeping, with electrodes already adhered to his chest. His family trailed behind, their faces pale with terror and disbelief. They had driven him here themselves, desperate to make it in time. And now they stood outside those doors, hoping for a miracle.

Inside that *resuscitation* room, chaos reigned. Nurses, *residents*, and *attendings* moved in a rehearsed dance, their roles well-defined. From my vantage point, I could only catch glimpses - arms moving swiftly, a *defibrillator* charging, syringes filled and emptied, voices overlapping with commands and confirmations. Though I was physically present, my mind kept slipping back to the scene across the hall. I couldn't help but wonder what was happening - had they achieved *Return of Spontaneous Circulation (ROSC)*? Was his heart beating again? Were the family's prayers being answered?

I couldn't see what happened next, but I knew that something had changed. Then, the doors finally opened. As they prepared to move him for further care (He was being wheeled out and back through the same doors he was rushed through), the doors opened wide, and I caught a full view of the room. It looked like a hurricane had passed through. Equipment lay scattered, wrappers and gloves littered the floor, and the bed was surrounded by remnants of a battle fought hard.

Taking my eyes off, I turned back to my mentor with a flurry of questions that he acknowledged with a nod and detailed explanations. Even though the chaos had finally settled, the lingering silence felt deafening, leaving my thoughts hovering between two rooms, two lives, and two outcomes. In those minutes, I had seen the very essence of what it meant to practice medicine - the relentless fight against disease, the hope that clings to even the smallest sign of life, and the understanding that sometimes, despite everything, the outcome is often beyond our control.

Moments like these carry a duality that I find hard to describe - a sense of triumph mingled with the weight of what could have been. That patient's heart had started beating again, but the memory of his lifeless form, the chaotic dash to revive him, and the uncertainty in his family's eyes remained etched in my mind. These were the moments that really put into perspective the kind of doctor I aspire to become.

Every day in the *ER* is a reminder of the fragility of life. It is a place where time seems to bend, stretching out in intense action and compressing in the aftermath. It's a place where the line between life and death is often blurred, where the outcome of a situation can shift in an instant. And it is in this space, amidst the chaos and calm, that the true meaning of wearing a white coat becomes clear. The weight of that coat is more than just fabric; it is the accumulation of every life we touch, every decision we make, every victory, and every loss. It is the burden of being both a healer and a witness to the endless cycle of life and death. Medicine, I learned that day, is not always the triumphant battle against disease we envision; sometimes, it is doing everything you can, and realising that control is often just an illusion.

Despite the challenges and horrors we witness, we often learn to appreciate what we have only after it's gone. This realisation makes us forget to be grateful for the chance to help and heal, a noble calling that not everyone is granted. This experience shaped me in ways I couldn't have imagined. It taught me that medicine is as much about the people we lose as it is about those we save. It revealed the human limitations of what we can and cannot do. Most importantly, it taught me that wearing that white coat means bearing witness to both hope and heartbreak, sometimes in the same breath.

IN THE SHADOW OF STILLNESS

Dr Maryam Rahmatullah and Dr Esra'a Alnaqeeb

I think a sliver of our faith in humanity evaporated that day. Who could commit such a heinous and despicable crime?

As we looked at the man, lifeless and limp in front of us, it felt as though life was draining from us alongside him. Every second seemed longer than the last, time stretching endlessly on as CPR continued.

He was a John Doe, brought in by *paramedics* with no pulse, blood dripping down the sides of the *gurney*. They found him on the street in a dark alleyway, with a gaping stab wound on his inner thigh. He looked young, possibly mid-twenties or mid-thirties. There was no identity card or way of knowing who he was or where he came from.

"Reassess!" The doctor's voice snapped me out of my daze.

Beep. Beep. Beep. They hooked some monitors onto him and used a strange machine to analyse his *vital signs.*

A minute passed.

Two.

"*PEA*!" they called out. Our eyes met; foreheads creased in confusion.

A quick Google search, filled with hopeful anticipation, showed us what those three letters meant.

"*Pulseless electrical activity (PEA)*"

His heart still wasn't beating.

At that moment, ours felt like they had stopped too.

We watched in horror, clutching each other's hands, leaning on one another for support, feeling as if we might collapse at any moment. Yet, the team continued their efforts to resuscitate his lifeless body.

The doctors behaved as though it was just another day at work – indifferent, cold, utterly desensitised. They laughed and cracked jokes, their voices piercing the gravity of the moment, a painful reminder of how detached they seemed. We couldn't quite make out what they were saying, but their smiles and nonchalant demeanour were unsettling. It was unfathomable. How could they behave this way? How could they treat this life-and-death struggle as if it were nothing more than another item on their checklist?

Yet.

Yet, their efficiency was undeniable. The team worked like clockwork - one managing the airway, another performing chest compressions, each fitting into their roles perfectly; where someone else stepped in, another tapped out, seamlessly taking over. They knew what they were doing.

It was almost surreal: the mechanical rhythm of their work, paired with their apparent lack of emotion. The scene left us torn between awe at their skill and disbelief at their seeming indifference.

As time dragged painfully on, the horror of the unsuccessful attempts bore down on us. The only one in the room who appeared to have the same reaction as the four of us was one of the younger-looking *paramedics* who had brought the patient in. He looked just as dazed and terrified, mirroring how we were feeling. The panic in his eyes and pallor of his face told us that this may be his first time witnessing an incident like this too.

"We'll give him this unit of blood and call it a day," the team leader called out. Blood was rushing to my head. My heart did a backflip in my chest.

"No!" we whispered to one another in unison, our hearts pounding in our chests. This can't be the end.

"Please, please, God, let him live. Let him live. Bring him back. Please," my friend whispered, her voice cracking as tears threatened to spill.

In the corner of my vision, I saw a police officer at the far end of the room, jotting something down on a sticky note. I wanted to see what he had written, but he was too far away.

"Reassess."

Still PEA

Still nothing.

I looked into the nurse's eyes and, at that moment, I understood. There was no coming back.

The doctor performed an *ultrasound* of his heart, just to be sure there was no movement. Everything was so still in that moment. And, most importantly, his heart – the one we had all hoped and prayed would miraculously start again, beat again, show any activity – was still. Nothing. Just stillness.

Then the team leader called the time of death, "10:18 p.m."

She thanked everyone for their efforts, and the crowd in the room began to dissipate.

It felt as if time froze at that moment.

I couldn't bear to look at anyone or anything. I was in a state of pure disbelief, shock, and grief. My eyebrows furrowed as I stared at the body in front of me, stripped from head to toe - dishevelled, exposed, lifeless. No one moved to cover him or to maintain his modesty. Not even a sheet of cloth. Nothing.

We were the only ones left in the room, alongside the same paramedic who had found the patient. He still looked pale.

Moments later, another police officer walked in, flashing his CID badge.

"Who's the doctor here?" he asked.

"N-no, no one. We're just students," we squeaked.

"All of you are students? No doctors?" he jokingly replied. We blinked at him and nodded our heads, trying to stay composed. The patient was still in my peripheral vision.

We lingered there for what felt like an eternity, just five to ten minutes in reality, frozen in disbelief, trying to grasp what we had just witnessed. Slowly, the weight of it all began to settle over us, crushing any sense of composure we had left. Shuffling out of the room and nudging each other, we scrambled out into the darkness of the car park outside the hospital.

We each grappled with the incident in our own way. My friend broke down and started sobbing uncontrollably, the sound of her cries filling the silence of the night. Others stood motionless, staring at the ground as if the enormity of the moment had paralysed them. I paced nervously, my hands trembling, still in denial, unsure of how to feel.

Hearing about tragedies and crimes like this on the news had always felt distant, a story removed from our reality. But this… this was different. We had seen someone's life slip away right in front of us. The finality of it, the sheer fragility of life, hit us in waves.

We now knew how it felt – not just to hear about death, but to witness it. It's something you can't unsee, a heartbreak that etches itself into your soul forever. We all coped in our own ways that day, but the weight of what we experienced is something we carry together – a bond born out of shared heartbreak.

FACING THE UNKNOWN

Dr Marwa Abdelmagid

It was my last year of medical school. I was so excited to finally experience what being a real doctor felt like - to step into the shoes of those I admired and finally find my place in this world. But then, everything changed. War broke out in my home country, Sudan. If you've ever heard about it, you know it's a place that's suffered. My university decided to relocate to Tanzania, a place I'd never even thought about before. To be honest, I had to look it up on the map when I got the email, just a glance at the few drastic changes the war forced us to make. If I wanted to continue my degree, I'd have to go there. That email marked the beginning of a new chapter, one that would change everything about me - how I saw the world, and how I felt about life. It wasn't just a turning point; it was the start of something entirely new.

Tanzania felt like a world apart. People were kind and willing to help, even though we couldn't speak their language, and only a few spoke English. Swahili wasn't hard, but I refused to learn it at the beginning because I didn't want to let go of who I was. I thought learning it meant changing how I think or how I feel. Fitting in was hard at first, but I'll never forget how they made us feel welcome. We weren't treated like strangers, at least not in the way other countries had treated my people. There were curious looks, yes, but overall, it was a place that embraced us, and that meant everything.

Dar es Salaam was the farthest I'd ever been from home alone. I was used to being sheltered, only allowed to stay over at my grandmother's house. Now I was in a foreign country, alone, with no family to fall back on, no familiar walls to comfort me. The loneliness was overwhelming. I couldn't handle even the simplest tasks - paying for electricity, buying groceries - things I'd never had to do alone before. But I had to learn. My family was counting on me. They were waiting for me to come back as a doctor, to make them proud. I had to fight, not just for my education, but for myself.

We soon began our hospital rotations. We tried to blend in, to be helpful wherever we could. I was desperate to learn, to gain every bit of knowledge and skill I could, so I could take it back home. I was always focused and always on the lookout for opportunities to grow. I arrived early, often before anyone else, and left late, sometimes as late as 10 p.m. I couldn't bear the thought of missing something important, of letting my family down by not giving my all. I was searching for a mentor, someone to guide me, to help me overcome my fears and to teach me what it truly meant to be a doctor. Eventually, I found him. He gave me advice and opportunities I couldn't have imagined. I'll forever be grateful to him. He didn't just teach me medicine; he showed me how to find myself.

Even as I immersed myself in my studies, doubts lingered. Have I seen enough? Learned enough about the people, their culture, and who they really were? Eight months later, when the chance came to move to another hospital to experience more, I hesitated. But my mentor's words echoed in my mind: "Face your fears." So, I took the leap.

When I began my next placement, from the very first day, it brought everything back. It felt like home - the same kind of setting, the same hospitality, the same atmosphere. It stirred up memories I thought I'd buried. I hadn't moved on; I had just pushed those memories away, not wanting to relive the darkness of war, the constant threat of being bombed, killed, or injured. Those were the reasons my family and I had left Sudan.

At first, I regretted the move. I asked my supervisor if I could go back, but that wasn't an option. So, I had to face my fears once more. And yet, here I learned more. The pressure felt different; it wasn't a competition anymore. I could learn at my own pace. But the event that would shatter me hadn't happened yet.

It was a Tuesday morning during our *ER* round. That's when I saw her - a little girl, barely a year old, severely dehydrated. A simple condition, but one that could turn deadly fast. The nurses struggled to find a vein to start an intravenous *(IV)* line. I watched as they tried over and over - nine times at least - each failed attempt leaving me more anxious. They tried her skull next, but nothing. A few of us suggested the *intraosseous (IO)* route, a common procedure back home for cases like this. But, as students, our voices were barely heard. We were at the bottom of the food chain.

The child's condition worsened. I thought they believed she was stable, but she wasn't even breathing. They moved on to the femoral vein, but still no monitors on her since another child with a heart condition occupied the bed. The ER was full. The doctor asked if anyone wanted to try the *femoral vein.* His eyes landed on me. I was just a student, never having done this before. But I didn't hesitate. I had never let an opportunity pass me by. I tried once and failed. On the second attempt, I managed to draw a small amount of blood, just 2 cc, not enough. The doctor tried three more times to get what was needed for the lab. All this time, the little girl was slipping away. Her skin turned ghostly pale, her body ice-cold, her eyes sunken in. Her mother stood by the wall, silent tears streaming down her face, clutching her twin brother in a pouch on her back. She looked helpless, knowing she had waited too long to bring her daughter to the hospital.

Finally, the head of the *ER* arrived. By then, the girl's breathing had stopped. The head doctor began *CPR*, pressing so hard that I could almost hear the ribs cracking. She shouted for *adrenaline*, but the syringe came too late. The girl's mother collapsed to the floor. One of the other patients' mothers picked up the twin, offering some comfort, as if giving the grieving mother space to absorb the impossible reality.

Moments later, I saw the head doctor stop CPR. I was stunned. Why did she stop? In the movies, they always keep going. They never give up, and the person comes back. But this wasn't a movie. The nurses, the doctors, all exchanged that look, the one that says, "We did everything we could." I glanced at the mother. She was running toward the doctor, begging in Swahili, pleading for her not to stop. I didn't know the language well, but I didn't need to. Her anguish was universal. A nurse tried to explain, saying they'd done all they could, but the mother wouldn't accept it. She began CPR herself, desperately pressing on her daughter's tiny chest, refusing to let go, refusing to lose her to the void.

After what felt like hours, but was only minutes, the mother collapsed, cradling her daughter's lifeless body with one hand while pounding the floor with the other. It was as if she were trying to dig a grave with her bare hands, or perhaps punish herself for what she saw as her failure.

I didn't know what to feel. Was it fear? Grief? I didn't know this child or her mother. I was lost, overwhelmed by emotions I couldn't name. It was the first time I had watched a soul leave a body, the first time I had witnessed a loved one's raw, unfiltered reaction to the finality of death. Despite being in this field for four and a half years, I had only seen these moments in movies, where you know, deep down, it's all just acting. But this wasn't a movie.

This was real, and there was no script, no makeup to wipe away, no going home to loved ones after the scene was over.

After witnessing the nurse carry the little girl away to an isolated room, giving her mother a moment to say her goodbyes and sparing the other mothers in the *ER* from the sight of her lifeless body, I felt numb. I walked down the hallway, my mind reeling, trying to make sense of what I'd just seen. Why did it have to happen? Could I have done something to save her? Isn't medicine supposed to be about saving lives? But we couldn't save her. What if it had been someone I cared about on that table? These questions buzzed in my mind, each one like a weight pressing down on my chest.

I found an empty chair by the door and sank into it, feeling like I was carrying the weight of the world on my shoulders. Moments later, the silence was shattered by the sound of a door slamming open. I looked up, and there she was - the little girl's mother. I'd recognise her anywhere now. She crumpled to the ground, her cries filling the hallway. Hospital staff and patients stood around her, silent, wearing expressions of helplessness and sorrow. They all had that same look - the look that said, I wish I could help you. I'm so sorry for your loss.

I wanted to go to her, to hold her, to tell her that her daughter had gone to a better place. But I couldn't move. I just sat there, paralysed, my thoughts spiralling. I couldn't stop thinking that this could have been me or someone I loved. It was like watching black dye spread through a glass of water, darkening everything in its path.

After a few minutes, some people came over to comfort her, offering what little solace they could. I felt a small wave of relief wash over me. I didn't know what to say, didn't know how to comfort her, didn't know how she felt because, deep down, I didn't. I couldn't.

As the bus rumbled along the crowded streets, my thoughts drifted back to that small ER room and the helplessness I had felt watching the little girl slip away. It wasn't the first time I'd seen suffering, but today felt different. It was as if something had cracked open inside me, revealing a truth I hadn't been prepared to face. I had entered medical school believing that, with enough knowledge and skill, I could save everyone - that becoming a doctor meant I would always know what to do, and that I'd be in control. But today's experience showed me just how fragile and unpredictable life really is.

I stared out of the window, watching the vibrant streets blur by. Life went on, and people moved about, unaware of the battle that had been lost just hours before. In that moment, I realised something profound: being a doctor wasn't about being a hero or always having the answers. It wasn't about being perfect or thinking we could cheat death. It was about standing at the edge of the unknown, facing the inevitable, and still doing everything in our power to make a difference.

EBBS AND FLOWS

Dr Srutdi Kamalam Natarajan

It was an unusually quiet morning in the ER. I could only think to myself because verbally addressing the tranquillity apparently summons chaos and gets the ER hustling. And as much as I love working, no one can resist the allure of a peaceful day at work. However, even if work is not as busy, we must keep patrolling the wards, go through case files, talk to patients, and learn more about their complaints. On most days, this process is as monotonous as it can get.

"Hey! Come hear this *pansystolic murmur*! I don't think I have ever heard this one before," my colleague calls out to me. I walk over to the patient, and after a brief introduction, I auscultate him.

And there - I heard it.

A *murmur* I have been reading about in my books for the past four years strikes clearly against my stethoscope. The quiet, continuous lull of the day breaks as fascination and gratitude fill me. There you go, another day, another challenge, and hopefully something new worth learning about. The feeling is almost like how one might feel if they encountered a celebrity on the streets. The same breathless excitement, as you put on a facade to remain calm.

That's the thing about hospital wards. Something happens and we all get swept up in its waves. Feet rushing, doctors whispering to each other, some of us are trying to save lives, the others like to take a backseat and observe, and some of us are looking for a moment to step away and close our eyes. The ER is rarely still, but there are moments where it can also feel lonely and quiet. Once the excitement subsides, the fabricated clinical peacefulness ensues until something happens again. And of course, it did. We heard the speakers blaring with an announcement, "*Code Blue* at A1 emergency!" The same patient had lost his pulse. The serene air quickly turned tense. The doors of the ER swung wide open, and the entire *resuscitation* team rushed in. "I cannot feel a pulse, starting chest compressions," the senior resident calls out. This was the very first time I got to witness the whole protocol. I watched hopefully, waiting for the resident to announce that he got a pulse.

We are taught to be healers. We are told to hope. So, a part of me truly believed that the patient would be okay because, till then, the portrayal of CPR in movies led me to believe that it always works. It turns out it's nothing like the movies. After several rounds of chest compressions, the resident moves away from the patient.

"Time of death - 10:11 a.m.," he says. I remember standing silently, soaking in the intensity of the whole situation and thinking, "The same heart that taught me earlier is no longer beating?" I watched the last breath of life leave someone's body helplessly. Two minutes is what we had to come to terms with it before the ER cleared out. Some of us have not processed what just happened. We watch as patients toss and turn on their respective beds, listening to the white noise provided by the heart monitors.

Doctors are always taught to be compassionate, kind and empathetic, but at the same time, they don't get the time or space to process their own emotions. Over time, we simply learn to compartmentalise our feelings because every patient deserves quality care, which is possible only if we feel our best, both physically and mentally. We have to make sure that whatever happens with one patient should never compromise care for another.

Some clinical symptoms are often described as waxing and waning, which simply means that the patient has complaints intermittently that seem to appear and resolve repeatedly. Maybe, it's a reminder that nothing is truly constant. Illness, the moon, our lives in medicine - everything is always shifting, and we need to move with the tide. It constantly waxes and wanes, but we know it truly never changes shape. Similarly, our journey is going to be filled with disappointments, recoveries, and miracles, but the purpose of being a doctor never changes.

The Unseen Miracles of Medicine

It was at the break of dawn when the staff rolled her in, and her family ran along anxiously. "Please help her," pleaded the man who held her hand. I remember watching the resident trying to wake her up, but she lay unresponsive. She was just around twenty years old and had unfortunately developed *infectious peritonitis* and *sepsis.*

I saw her fight for survival. She held on for as long as she could as we hooked her up to the ventilator. We are often called 'miracle workers.' I am always forced to ask, Where is the miracle? Because only a miracle could save her at this point, and I have been here long enough to know that one was not coming. It wasn't long until I watched her monitor flash a flat line.

However, towards the end of the very same shift, I recollect my colleague narrating her experience with a very old woman, around eighty years old, who had come into the hospital with severe breathlessness and multiple comorbidities. She was immediately evaluated, and within a few hours of starting medications, she was sitting up comfortably and having casual conversations with the staff.

In one day, I saw a twenty-year-old slip away and an eighty-year-old regain her strength. Maybe that was the miracle. Not every treatment ensures survival. That is the bitter truth. But medicine is not measured only in victories. It is in the effort - the unrelenting pursuit of healing, even when the outcome is out of our hands. Our best efforts might not always feel rewarded, but the gratification arises from the fact that we are committed to the delivery of our best care and expertise at every given opportunity.

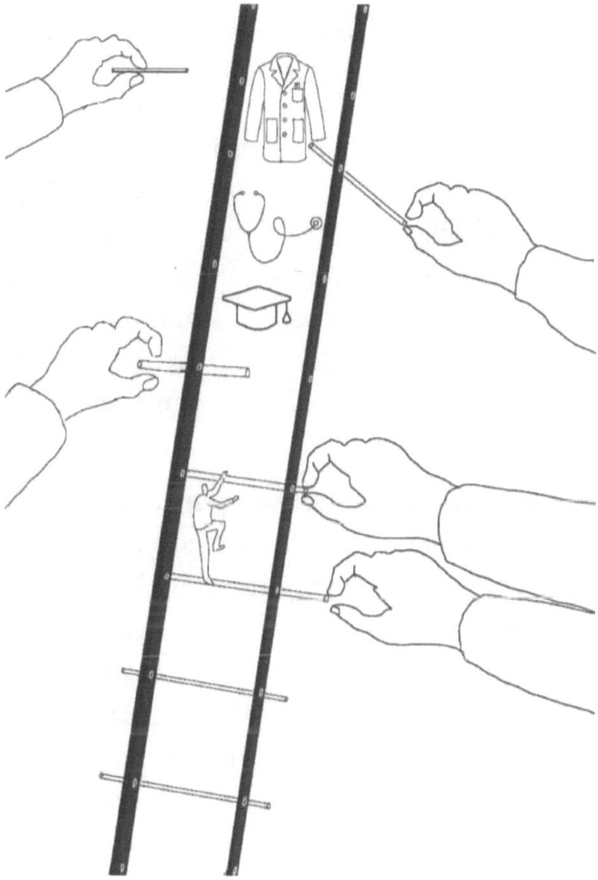

ASPIRATIONS AND ADVICE

FROM DREAMS TO DIAGNOSIS

Dr Aiman Hidayat

It all started after my twelfth exams when I was deciding on my career path, and suddenly, the thought of medicine crossed my parents' minds. We then researched and decided on Pakistan as the place for me. I still remember it being a hot, sunny day during *Ramadan* when I had my flight to Pakistan, and my mother came to drop me off at the dorm. My heart was sinking, and my eyes were full of tears as I bid farewell to my family and embarked on this journey.

Each day left a nostalgic effect on my mind as I moved through the steps of my white coat expedition to becoming a medical professional, which was a transformative odyssey replete with twists and turns that tested my resolve, fostered resilience, and ultimately shaped me into a compassionate and skilled individual. I embarked on my white coat journey, leaving behind the comfort of my familiar surroundings in the UAE, to pursue a medical career in Pakistan, as it marked a broadening of my perspective and forever altered the trajectory of my life. The transition was complex as I had to adapt to the stark contrast in facilities, cultural norms, and environment between the UAE and Pakistan.

My initial step was applying for the *entrance examination*, and then I took a detour, embarking on a winding path that led me to the dorms. The interior of the dorm reminded me that success cannot be achieved within a comfort zone; one must venture into challenges and embrace trials to grow. While I acknowledge that pursuing a career in medicine was initially driven by my parents' wishes, I must admit that I have grown to like the field, and now this thought aligns with my own interests and goals.

Despite the challenges in terms of accommodation, food, and study environment, I began my preparation for the entrance test. Focusing on my studies and staying committed to my goals. Due to a completely different course of the test and limited time as the day of the exam approached, I felt increasingly nervous. Unfortunately, I failed my first attempt, and even though I did get some university offers, the high fee demands made me step back and rethink my decision.

My father was having sleepless nights, wondering how he would fulfil the highly demanding fees of the universities. However, due to a payment he had yet to receive, he realised he wouldn't be able to do so, and that pushed him to lead a stressful lifestyle. So, I decided with a heavy heart that this is not the end of the world, and if I want, I can still achieve my dreams. The disappointment of failure was palpable, and self-doubt crept in, threatening to derail my dreams. However, I refused to let failure define me, and with unwavering determination, I regrouped, reassured, and prepared again for the exam. After one whole year of dedication and hard work, I attempted again. But this time too, the hurdles were set again, the test was cancelled multiple times, and each cancellation felt like a blow to my morale.

My test centre was in another city, so the night before the test, we decided to start our journey towards a city called Haripur. Although we reached there the night before the test, all the hotels were surprisingly full. This was because many aspirants like me had come earlier too. To our surprise, we couldn't find a place to stay for the night, and one of my uncle's faraway friends decided to give us shelter in their village. As we approached their house, the night became darker, and when we reached, we found out there was no electricity. The whole night, my mom was giving me air with a hand fan so I could sleep peacefully. The morning of the test, I woke up early, prayed, and set off on the journey towards the centre. At the centre, while we were waiting for the papers to be distributed, it started pouring heavily. As a result, the test got cancelled, and all the candidates went back home disappointed.

A new test date was set, and once again the journey began. I worked harder than before, and this time we set off on the road again towards the test centre. The test went well, and I came out happy and started the ride back home. On the way back, we received the message that the test paper had been leaked, and that's why it is now rescheduled to a new date. Wow, now that's a turn of events. I was burnt out; I couldn't look at the books anymore, and the walls of my room were feeling more like a jail. The time of the test kept coming closer, and I was getting lazier. Just one week before the test, I decided to stop wasting time and regain all the knowledge. The test went well this time, and hopefully no more hurdles.

I struggled to maintain my motivation, and there were times when I felt like giving up. But I refused to let my dreams slip away. Finally, the day of the result came; my hands were shaking, and my heart was throbbing so fast I thought it would jump off my chest. Finally, I had passed my exam, but my journey was far from over, even though I had gotten a seat in the best university of my dreams. The main challenge of surviving through five years of med school was yet to be surpassed.

The five years that followed were a kaleidoscope of experiences, a vibrant tapestry woven from threads of challenge, growth, and self-discovery. During my five years of medical studies, I encountered individuals from diverse backgrounds. While some became friends, others proved to be deceitful. Through these experiences, I learned valuable lessons about human nature. I even acquired proficiency in various languages, broadening my communication skills and fostering a deeper understanding of the culture and traditions of Pakistan. As I delved deeper into the world of medicine, the intricacies of the human body revealed themselves to me like a masterpiece of art. The precision of surgery, the nuance of diagnosis, and the empathy of patient care. Each aspect was a brush stroke on the canvas of my expertise. I devoured knowledge, attending lectures, participating in discussions, and engaging in hands-on training.

Five years of med school passed by so quickly, and staying away from home made me realise the importance of family. Also, the new people I met in my life created an impact on my personality and shaped it beautifully.

The thrill of discovery coursed through my veins like adrenaline, propelling me forward upon completing my studies. I embarked on my *internship* at a teaching hospital, a crucible of real-world experience. The wards, a kaleidoscope of human suffering and resilience, tested my mettle, forcing me to confront the complexities of healthcare. I worked alongside seasoned professionals, learning from their expertise and contributing my own skills, shaped by years of dedication. Now, I am taking proactive steps towards specialisation by applying for programmes in foreign countries that will provide me with diverse perspectives, advanced training, and wider career opportunities.

THE SOUNDTRACK OF MEDICAL SCHOOL

Hurairah Faatimah Muzammil

Medical school is not just a test of the best memorisation skill, but also a training exercise teaching you to adapt and learn from every patient. From the *auscultation* sounds heard through a *stethoscope* to the eerie silence of a *cadaver*, each experience is bound to leave you grappling with profound lessons.

Our journey of learning started with our silent teachers - the cadavers - who taught us the various elements of anatomy and made us marvel at the detailed and extensive design of the human body. I still remember making my first cautious cut with the *scalpel* on the thorax, so focused that I could hear the scalpel make the incision. While the dissection room boomed with excited yet nervous chatter, all I heard was the cut piercing through layers of skin and fat, easing out into muscle. In the sessions that followed, the sound of bone whirring as we cut through the ribs and the sounds of internal organs being handled made us fall in love with *anatomy*, even as the lengthy hours persisted.

One of my professors, Dr A, always expressed the importance of the skill of listening, be it to the patient or the numerous sounds we learn throughout our medical school life. Moving from cadavers to real-life humans seemed like a bigger transition than from one year to the next. With living humans and no imaging or operations, all we could rely on was the history our patients gave us and the skills we possessed. Starting off with the cardiovascular block, we were exposed to the famous "lub-dub" of our hearts and soon transitioned to *murmurs*, *heaves*, and *thrills*. With the following blocks came *palpation* and *percussion*, adding more sounds for our minds to absorb. For what our mind doesn't know, our eyes cannot see, or in this case, our ears cannot hear.

Every examination skill we learned, another sound made itself known as a key diagnostic indicator. With each passing interaction, I learned that the art of listening does not just mean hearing, but also extends to the signs and symptoms patients experience. The challenges of listening were many. From identifying missed sounds to differentiating murmurs from different variants, I was taught the importance of precision and focus.

I remember the struggle I faced in identifying an *S4* vs an *aortic stenosis murmur*. Oh, and the *crepitations* and *crackles* made me question life. But through these experiences, I learned that the body always speaks to you. It presents you with every sound and symptom. However, it is the diagnostic skill of a doctor that contributes to accurate assessment and appropriate treatment.

Dr E, in one of her first lectures, told us, "The body always answers; it is the right questions that it seeks." That has always motivated me to look for signs and be alert for both the rarest and the commonest diagnoses.

The art of sound goes a step further and teaches us to focus on verbal and non-verbal communication from a patient. To truly listen to a patient is to immerse oneself in their story, paying attention not only to what is said but also to how it is said. The tone of their voice, the pacing of their words, and the pauses between sentences often carry as much significance as the content itself. A hesitance to answer could hint at discomfort or fear, while a hurried explanation might signal anxiety. Beyond words, there are the silent cues - the shifting of posture, the fleeting expressions, or the way their hands tremble as they gesture. These subtleties often reveal what words cannot, offering insight into the patient's emotional and physical state.

For instance, a patient who cannot articulate their pain due to neurological impairment might communicate their distress through facial expressions, restless movements, or avoidance of touch. Learning to hear these silent messages is as crucial as mastering any medical device.

Medical school teaches you to fine-tune your hearing - not just for sounds, but for meaning. You realise that every patient has a unique soundtrack, and it is your job to listen carefully. Whether it's the rhythm of a heartbeat or the tremor in a voice, these sounds are windows into the human experience. It teaches us to distinguish between the mundane and extraordinary, instilling in us that listening is not just a diagnostic tool, it is a connection to the pulse of life itself.

DEAR FELLOW DOCTORS

Dr Amna Ibrahim Zaidan

To my dearest junior doctors and medical students, I promise that you will overcome this - *In Sha Allah* (God willing).

This, too, shall pass.

Always remember that.

Trust and believe in yourself.

You have accomplished so much and reached so far because you are competent, because you are you, and nobody else.

The shadow of self-doubt that followed you ever since you were preparing to get into medical school will, unfortunately, keep following you. The good news is that you will be able to deal with it better. It will not overpower you anymore.

Give it time.

You will be more in control of your life. The more mountains you have to climb, the easier it will be to expect difficulties, and the easier it will be to prepare for each journey. They may be different mountains, but the process is all the same. Years from now, I promise that you will look back and laugh rather than cry.

To some of you, I might sound like I'm overreacting or dramatising medical school or the medical journey in general. But the truth is, your mental health is more important than any grade you receive, any scolding remarks you hear, or any day you procrastinate. The reason? Because in medicine, your self-esteem will be challenged repeatedly by doctors, by patients, and even by colleagues and friends. And in those moments, **you will be your**

only defence. In clinical rotations, rocks will be thrown at you everywhere you go. You will need to learn how to dodge them, how to catch them, and how to overcome them.

"Number one rule is Respect."

Oh, the number of times you'll hear that one. It's nothing bad, of course. It's common sense in the medical field where teamwork is expected. But you know what's not common sense and what's not talked about? Creating boundaries. Drawing lines. **Respecting yourself first**.

You need to recognise when someone - a doctor, patient, or colleague - is crossing the line and being disrespectful. That's when your self-worth and self-respect need to be protected, and their behaviour needs to be addressed. Don't be intimidated. **You paid to be there, and you deserve to be there**. No one can tell you otherwise. This is a crucial period where your "doctor personality" is forming. You'll be faced with many difficulties, insults, and mistreatments as you go on this journey, so you need to set boundaries and draw lines early on to help you recognise ill treatment and deal with it better.

With each rotation, we go to different hospitals, which could be private or governmental hospitals. We also deal with different medical staff, different doctors, nurses, and patient demographics. This is challenging to our mental health and to our personality. Our dear introverts probably have a hard time learning new social skills, while extroverts among us struggle with their unique self-expression being spotlighted and criticised. Don't worry, we've all been there, done that. Time heals all wounds, so make mistakes and be proud of them. That is the only way you will genuinely have important lessons embedded in you. You are not a robot who is meant to be smiling twenty-four-seven while greeting every medical staff member with overwhelming energy just so that they have a good first impression of you. So, what if they don't? You will be told to change who you are so that others may like you better. But, **don't fall into that trap**. It's advice rooted in insecurity, not goodwill. **Be yourself.** Not arrogant, not selfish, **but confident and genuine.** When you stay true to who you are, you will naturally communicate with respect, and in turn, you will earn the respect of others.

Expect setbacks and disappointments. But also **expect that you will become a better person.** Some moments will make you feel like crawling into a hole from embarrassment. Trust me, we've all been there.

On my first day in *Obstetrics and Gynaecology (OBGYN)* rotation as a medical student, I was excited to be involved in *history* taking from a new mother who had just undergone a normal delivery. As a result, I ended up abruptly asking her during the conversation if she had any sexually transmitted diseases.

Needless to mention, both the mother and her husband were baffled, staring at me (yes, her husband was right there). The supervising doctor hit the brakes on the interview and later explained to me that this question is either asked indirectly by asking about symptoms or at least in a private and confidential manner.

During my *Direct Observation Clinical Encounter Examination (DOCEE)* exam in the *OBGYN* rotation, I was assigned to a patient who had just undergone a normal delivery. While taking history, I repeatedly asked the patient why she had undergone a Caesarean section. In my defence, I was pretty nervous. The mother, however, was kind enough to clarify each time. Then, I went on to confidently ask her that if she had a delivery, then where was the newborn baby? The newborn was right in front of me in the crib.

These moments may haunt you now, but one day, they'll be the stories you laugh about with your colleagues. You are meant to make mistakes. They don't define you. But if you reflect and learn from them, your wisdom will shape you into the doctor you wish to be.

Now, let me give you a hard truth:

You will most definitely get scolded for not introducing yourself. It's a magical spell cast on us, medical students. We introduce ourselves with an artificial smile (even with barely four hours of sleep the night before), so that we have a good first impression on our evaluators and to develop "doctor social skills," making us polite and professional team players.

So, why do we forget to introduce ourselves? It could be burnout. It could be being overwhelmed by our environment. It could be the fact that we change hospital settings and rotations so frequently that we get tired of it, or we get used to being part of the team so naturally that we unknowingly skip the formalities.

Once in my *Internal Medicine* rotation, I went into a patient's room following a doctor and saw that the patient was already having a serious conversation with the doctor, which made me hesitant to interrupt for a self-introduction. I regretted it instantly when the doctor humiliated me in front of the patient. I can say it was a teaching experience until he started pointing a finger at me (poking my glasses and forehead) with no personal space while "teaching" me about the ethics of introducing myself.

Criticism is essential for growth, **but only when it's constructive.** Feedback helps us improve, but **mistreatment is**

never acceptable. Feedback is valuable for medical students to grow as better doctors and perhaps as better humans. This stops when limits are crossed.

My dear medical students, you are not inferior to anyone. You are not the bottom of the food chain. Do not let anyone, no matter who it is, disrespect you. You are as valuable and important as the consultants in the hospital. No less. And always remember, **if you magnify the image of a person in your mind, you will unconsciously minimise yourself in their presence.**

All medical schools are different, but if you are given the choice to choose between rotating alone vs with a partner, I'd encourage you to choose someone you are acquainted with rather than a friend. It could give you company if you can't stand eating alone, for example (like me). You'll have lots of free time, too. In my opinion, I would encourage you to avoid choosing friends. It's work, not personal life, which means you'll have arguments due to differences on how you'd rather spend your time and in making several decisions. It's better to have someone you think will be a good work partner who will respect your individual decisions and not depend on you.

Finally, medical school will challenge you in ways you never imagined. But through it all, **believe in yourself.** You are here because you deserve it.

You will make mistakes. You will be embarrassed. You will feel lost at times. But in every moment of doubt, **remember why you started.**

One day, you won't just survive medical school. You will thrive.

And when you look back, you will realise you weren't just learning to become a doctor,

You were learning to become you.

THE JOURNEY OF MEDICAL LIFE

Dr Muzammil Hafeez

Doing medicine requires the skill of lifelong learning. To become successful doctors, we need to gather knowledge from teachers, seniors, patients, and our books. The world of medicine is an ocean of knowledge that is ever-changing. As doctors, we always need to update our knowledge. However, there are some things that form the cornerstone of the work that we do and some skills that never change.

I fondly remember one memory with my *ENT* professor, Dr Ram. As we stood in the operating theatre, he gave me advice before the start of our *tonsillectomy* operation on that day. He said, "You may be the best doctor with the best skills, but the most important aspect of our practice is communication with the patient." I took his advice to heart. And when I look through the journey of my medical practice, even today, this has not changed, and this will never change. I want every young doctor to learn and practice this.

Similarly, I remember an encounter with my *Paediatrics* professor, who taught me to always practise and deal with our patients with a smile. These things go a long way in building a healthy and trusting relationship with your patient.

When you treat a patient with compassion, the whole family trusts you. In my first week of my post-graduation in *Paediatrics* in *emergency*, I had a baby with *meningitis*. I had the opportunity to arrange for the baby's complete treatment, and the baby, at discharge, was completely normal. Later, the mother returned, this time not for her baby's problem but her problem, even though

I was a *paediatrician*. I then directed her to the appropriate doctor. This shows the impact of the trust built and the importance of respect and care when dealing with our patients.

As we go ahead through our medical practice, I hope we can all echo kindness and communication. Treating our patients does not only involve treating their disease, but also providing mental support, reassurance, and good counselling. Always remember - to you, it may be another day at work, but for that patient, you are the person saving their life and helping them out with their problem.

EXCELLENCE AND DIGNITY

Dr Tasnima Tayb

These are words of excellence, endeavour, and expectation that I have written and cello-taped to my table – a culmination of advice from some of the greatest doctors I have had the opportunity to learn from.

"It's not enough that you become a doctor – you have to take the best of each of us and accumulate it into your practice."

"I don't want you to simply guess; I want you to be confident in your knowledge. You have to be a good doctor. There's no way around it."

"Whenever you make a judgement, ensure that it is you who has seen it first-hand. You have seen the vitals. You have seen the patient. You have read the CT scan. Your decision, your eyes, your ears. I have been burnt many times relying on someone else's alone; now I make sure to verify from my side before proceeding."

"You have to be as reliable as a tool, no one second-guesses it."

"Whatever decision you make, always ask: how does it change my management? What value will it give me?"

"You cannot develop tunnel vision; if you don't think of it, you will miss it."

"The only interest is the best interest of the patient."

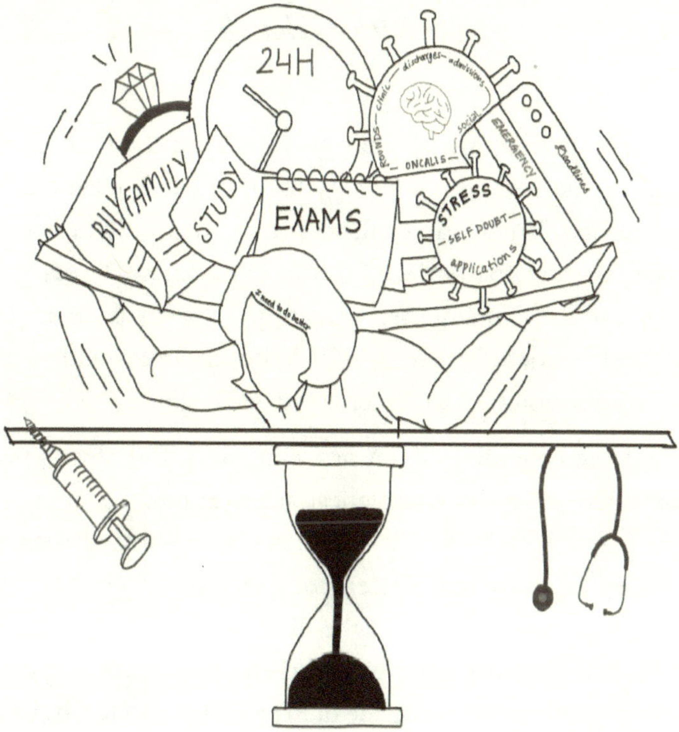

BURNOUT, BALANCE AND RESILIENCE

THE WEIGHT OF THE WHITE COAT

Dr Rita Alkhatib

I remember wearing my lab coat awkwardly for the first time as a foundation student, with a biology book in hand, feeling like I'd conquered life. When the truth was that I had only just learned that "oto" refers to the "ear." Little did I know, I was still as insignificant as a kindergarten student playing dress up, and that unspeakable pride of wearing your lab coat comes with a much greater responsibility than I ever could've imagined.

From the beginning of my academic days, I've always been a top achiever, more like the highest achiever in every task, every subject, extracurricular activity, etc. Thus, being among the crème de la crème of those students entering medical school had always been a given default, as I thought all it took to excel in this field was a love for science, good memory, and hard work. Of course, the marvellous field of medicine didn't take long to teach me how I was all wrong.

Here, everyone is smart, everyone is hard-working, and everyone has a memory made of steel. Yet, medicine is much more than that. Those who excelled were those who were able to heal, not practice; those who could connect dots, not tunnel vision; those who practised with the eye of a hawk, yet with hands of silk, a heart of a mother, and the mind of a righteous judge (a quote adapted from one of the sharpest and toughest surgeons whom I had the privilege of training under).

I soon learned that learning my books was not nearly close enough to real medicine. It was rather being in the clinical setting, learning about patients as humans rather than just isolated clinical pictures. I understood both the blessing and immense responsibility of being trusted with a patient's deepest private matters and of guarding their most vulnerable moments. We are in this setting not only practitioners but also trustees, advisers, and protectors.

There is a chasm between learning medicine and practising it. As students, we are conditioned to see patients as "cases" - a puzzle of symptoms to solve. But to the person lying in the hospital bed, they are much more than a clinical scenario. They are humans who, often for the first time in their lives, are revealing their most intimate fears and vulnerabilities. They don't understand the jargon that flows so easily from our mouths. They don't know the prognosis or the intricacies of the disease like we do. All they know is that something is wrong with their body, and they have placed their trust in us, hoping we can make it right.

I remember being asked to examine a patient on one of my first clinical days. It was a routine task, nothing out of the ordinary. But for me, it felt like climbing a mountain. My hands trembled, unsure of where to begin or how much pressure to apply. The patient, a middle-aged man with a weary but kind expression, noticed my hesitation.

With a gentle smile, he said, "You can't touch a patient with shaky hands. Those hands should be the cure. The moment you touch your patient is the moment his healing begins."

His words hit me like a bolt of lightning.

Medicine was not just about diagnosing diseases and prescribing treatment. It was about connecting, about the trust that begins the moment our hands meet theirs. In that brief encounter, I realised the importance of empathy and human connection in medicine. The patient didn't just need me to be knowledgeable; he needed me to be present, steady, and reassuring. For him, the encounter with me was a significant moment, one that would stay with him long after I left the room. But to me, it was just another clinical task in a long day of learning.

That moment taught me a valuable lesson: what may seem like a fleeting, routine interaction to us as medical professionals is often a pivotal experience for the patient. We might see dozens of patients in a day, but to each of them, that brief meeting is a memory that can shape their journey of healing. It's a reminder that we aren't just treating bodies - we are caring for minds and souls as well.

The importance of empathy in medicine cannot be overstated. When we approach a patient with cold detachment, focusing solely on the clinical aspects of their condition, we lose sight of the very essence of healing. Patients aren't just cases to be solved; they are individuals, each with their own unique fears, hopes, and uncertainties. And often, they are navigating an uncharted territory, unsure of what lies ahead. While we, as medical professionals, may grow accustomed to seeing disease, pain, and suffering on a daily basis, for them, this is their first time experiencing such vulnerability.

When a patient sits in front of us, they are not just asking for a diagnosis or a prescription. They are seeking understanding, reassurance, and guidance through an often frightening and unfamiliar process. This is why correct empathy and communication are so vital in medicine. It is not enough to be a brilliant diagnostician or a skilled surgeon. True healing begins with the connection we establish with our patients - the trust we build, the compassion we show, and the empathy we extend.

So, remember that while you might have an unpleasant face because you haven't had your lunch, the expression and tone of your voice can change their view on life. While it has gone unnoticed for you, they are not used to being undressed in front of strangers. While you might forget in a minute, they will remember for life.

FROM BURNOUT TO BALANCE

Dr F Hana Naushad

How would I survive medical school? This question flooded my mind and search history upon receiving my acceptance letter. I remember staring at the acceptance email; my heart was pounding from a mix of excitement and relief of finally getting accepted to medical school. The relief of achieving a dream I had worked long and hard for was soon overtaken by the fear of whether I would survive medical school. Everyone knows medical school is tough - it's a sacrifice of endless studying and sleepless nights, with a non-existent social life.

To add fuel to the fire, the lasting impact of the COVID-19 pandemic on the delivery of education left me even more fearful of what was to come. The shift to online learning and the uncertainty of clinical rotations and simulations made me question how prepared I would be for real-world practice.

As I now stand on the cusp of graduating, I look back with gratitude for the experiences that have shaped me. Medical school was more than just an academic journey. Looking back, I realise now that medical school was a journey of resilience, strength, and kindness. It was about learning to care for others as well as yourself. The challenges we faced were real, but so were the moments of joy, celebration, and achievements. To future medical students, I offer my reflections in hopes that they may guide and inspire you on your own journey.

The COVID-19 pandemic added an unexpected layer of complexity to an already challenging journey. Face-to-face lectures were replaced with online learning, and navigating this new change forced me to adapt quickly, emphasising the importance of flexibility in medical education. It was my first day of medical school. I entered the Zoom meeting of my lectures; I was overwhelmed by the sheer volume of information presented that day and the days that followed. The PowerPoint presentations seemed endless, and the virtual faces staring back at me reflected the same mix of excitement and anxiety that I was feeling. The first Anatomy lab focused on the *femur* bone. It felt like a whirlwind of unfamiliar terms as we explored the femur's intricate features from the *epicondyles* to the *fossae* to the important lines where muscles attach.

Faced with an avalanche of information, I knew I had to refine my study strategies. I discovered the power of active learning, incorporating techniques like spaced repetition and teaching concepts to my peers. Creating a structured schedule allowed me to allocate time efficiently, ensuring I covered all necessary material while avoiding burnout.

As I adapted to hybrid learning and the start of clinical rotations, and kept up with the relentless demands, I realised the need to prioritise my well-being by learning that caring for others begins with caring for myself first. After six months of no academic pressure due to the COVID-19 pandemic, being suddenly immersed in the chaos of medical school, from back-to-back lectures to constant exam pressure, was surely overwhelming. The burnout I experienced was beyond anything I'd anticipated about the realities of medical school. Throughout my journey, I faced countless situations that resulted in sleepless nights, social isolation, poor nutrition, and lack of physical activity - all of which had lasting physical, emotional, and social effects.

Amidst this relentless pace, I quickly learned that neglecting my self-care was neither sustainable nor conducive to efficiency.

Incorporating regular exercise – or as I like to call it, my mental health walks – a more balanced diet, and prioritising quality time with my family and friends, eventually became essential parts of my routine. Contrary to popular belief, taking the time to implement self-care practices that rejuvenated me allowed me to approach my academics and rotations with renewed energy and focus.

In high-stakes environments such as medical school, the value of friendship and support became increasingly clear to me. The friends I have in medical school today have allowed me to become the person that I am. Together, we tackled complex topics and tasks that often felt overwhelming when faced alone. Late-night study sessions transformed into collaborative learning experiences where we could share insights, clarify doubts, share resources, and motivate each other to keep pushing forward. Practising together for every *OSCE* exam became a must that not only improved our clinical skills but also built our confidence. These efforts not only made me feel less alone in a rigorous programme but also deepened the connection with my friends, who went from being peers to lifelong friends who understood the unique challenges that we faced.

While my friends in medical school were a pillar of support, the encouragement and love of my family and non-medical friends provided a comforting anchor outside the academic world. My parents' unwavering encouragement and belief in my abilities fuelled my determination during the most challenging times. Their constant support created a nurturing environment that allowed me to focus on my studies and personal growth. Their constant love and assistance reminded me that I was not alone on this journey, and it reinforced my will to persevere through any obstacle. Regular phone calls, video chats, and occasional visits with my loved ones offered comfort and a much-needed respite from academic pressures. Engaging in conversations and activities unrelated to medicine allowed me to decompress and recuperate.

In essence, building and growing relationships, both within and outside of medical school, were instrumental in my journey. They provided a sense of community and togetherness that made the challenges of medical school not only manageable but also enriching. I learned that my success was not my effort alone, but through the strength and support of those around me, and it shaped me into a more compassionate and well-rounded individual.

As I approach the end of my medical school era, I reflect on the lessons I've learned along the way: the importance of resilience, self-care, and the unbreakable support of loved ones. To those embarking on this demanding yet rewarding journey, remember that it's okay to ask for help and lean on others. Build a strong support network, prioritise your mental and physical well-being, and hold on to the passion that led you here. There will be challenges along the way; embrace them as they will prepare you for a fulfilling career in medicine.

HOLDING THE LIGHTNING WITHIN

Dr Anaam Parveen

Walking into medicine as the first in my family, I thought I had some idea of what lay ahead. Spoiler alert: I didn't. There's no guide or pep talks strong enough to brace you for what's coming. The struggle? It's real. The hustle culture? Though I liked it, even more real. But here's the thing, no one warns you about the mental rollercoaster, the kind that sneaks up on you in the middle of an endless, sleepless night. Or about how the growth you're supposed to experience while figuring out life in your late teens to early twenties now takes place in this high-pressure canister, reshaping you day by day. And every long night, there's this unspoken challenge hanging in the air: Are you going to make it through to the other side, or will this break you first?

Growth in medicine doesn't just happen; it demands pieces of you, tearing apart old assumptions and layering on new realities. By the second year, you realise that it's not just about learning facts or mastering techniques; it's like you're sprouting new leaves, while letting others fall and crumble to dust - only to feed off them.

The relentless studying hours don't just wear on you – they change you. You start seeing things through a sharper lens, and the once-clear boundary between theory and life begins to blur by your third year. It's still fine in the classroom, but step out, and suddenly, everything you only learned about has textures and physical elements.

Then, by my fourth year, it happened: my lightning-strike moment - the kind of realisation that leaves a scar, as unmistakable as if it had etched itself onto my skin. Fractal and unforgiving scar, weaving across skin in a jagged, chaotic map. Each forked branch resonated an echo of the impact, seared in as a mark of survival I'd carry permanently, whether or not I wanted to.

A brutal awakening to what it truly means to know. And that's the thing about knowledge: it's beautiful, until it isn't. Because now, with every glance, I saw the harsh truths that medicine revealed - the kind that turns your loved ones into case studies you never wanted. It's not just awareness, it's hyperawareness, and it doesn't let go. It clings to you and forces you to look deeper until all you can see are vulnerabilities that you're helpless to shield them from.

They joke about *'medical student syndrome'* as if it's some quirky phase – a rite of passage where you start diagnosing yourself with every rare disease in the textbooks. And maybe, knowing that might have saved me from falling into that trap. But this was something else, something darker. My mind didn't turn inward; it turned outward, catching on my parents, my family. That's the brutal cost of understanding. The very thing I'd once wanted, this ability to see and understand, had now turned on me. I had to carry it, whether I was ready or not. The deeper I looked, the more that scar etched itself into my life, reminding me of the truth I could never unsee.

Suddenly, it was like I'd put on X-ray glasses no one warned me about. The kind that won't get off me. My parents weren't just my parents anymore - they were walking medical puzzles, and every little complaint kicked off a mental diagnostic checklist. Mom mentions, "I've been getting these headaches..." and instantly, I'm running through possibilities from dehydration to something straight out of a medical horror show. When Dad decides to tell me, "My shoulder hurts since…" I'm in my head ruling out everything from a simple strain to conditions that would make even an experienced senior doctor break out in a sweat. Every cough, every ache, every harmless complaint from my parents set off an internal alarm, like I was a doctor on-call twenty-four-seven without the pay cheque.

Worse, I couldn't just focus on new symptoms; I was also running their past diagnoses in the background like an invisible file folder, asking myself, "Could this be related?" or "Does that explain it?" My brain was on constant overdrive, ticking off boxes, ruling things in and out. I'd turned into a one-person diagnostic lab that never shuts down.

Having this unasked-for X-ray vision superpower was doing wonders for my peace - and by wonders, I mean etching that lightning scar a little deeper every time. My parents took their medications with the trust of loyal patients, and while I believed in their doctors, my newfound "superpower" had other plans. Every tablet came with a hidden catalogue of risks, only I seemed to notice, like an ever-present fine print that wouldn't leave my sight.

It's funny, in a dark way - the more I understood, the less I could find comfort. My lightning scar flared up each time, as if reminding me that this awareness wasn't just a "gift" - it was a shadow.

Over time, however, the awareness dulled like the sound of rain on a long, dreary day. In the initial years, every symptom and every medication was a loud, persistent downpour that was impossible to ignore. But eventually, it all became one of those 'focus rainfall background sound,' the steady rhythm of medicine blending into life. Yet, every so often, a single drop would slip past the umbrella I tried to hold over myself - a symptom here, a newly prescribed pill there - each one landing with a startling clarity, soaking into me where it fell. Sharp and cold. No matter how quiet the rain became, that one drop would strike with a vividness that cut through numbness, stirring the ache of that lightning scar buried within.

Somewhere along the way, I found myself nudging everyone towards supplements and skincare, like I was patching up tiny cracks in the hope the whole thing might hold together. Vitamin D, Omega-3, a multivitamin here and there - it felt like I was making little bargains with fate, as if these tiny tablets were enough to keep bigger fears at bay. And they never questioned it. If anything, I saw a newfound trust they had in me. Maybe they just found it easier to humour me. Either way, I kept at it, slipping them "insurance" pills like I was building a fortress, one tablet at a time. At this rate, I'd probably have enough vitamins stockpiled to start my own pharmacy by next year.

But the hyperawareness didn't stop with my immediate family. Relatives started sending me their test results, labs, diagnoses – each one coming through me as if I were the family's unofficial gatekeeper of medical updates. It was like they trusted me to see things they couldn't, passing along their scans and reports like they were secrets I'd somehow know how to handle. Being the only one in medicine, I suppose they felt I was the safest pair of eyes. Each message was a reminder that illness had a way of weaving its way through everyone, and my mind would immediately begin its familiar routine of interpreting, analysing, and bracing for impact.

Knowing exactly how my parents' medical conditions were chipping away at them became its own kind of silent torment. Each diagnosis wasn't just a label; it was a slow, insidious erosion that only I seemed to see unfolding. I watched as the illnesses crept forward, inch by inch, quietly taking pieces of them, each symptom like a whisper of something slipping further out of reach. It was as if I were the only one holding onto the full weight of it, the one tethered to a truth that I wished I could ignore but couldn't unsee.

Yet, for all the weight this awareness carried, there was something to be grateful for: I could finally make sure my family and loved ones weren't just drifting through the system, vulnerable to oversights or misjudgements. Knowing I could be a safeguard for them, a little safety key they could count on, felt like a purpose woven into the burden. It gave me a sense of agency, of quiet reassurance that I could shield them in ways they might never even realise. And yet, even with this comfort, the fears lingered, quieter now, settling like shadows in the background. They've become familiar, like a heartbeat just beneath the surface, a reminder that some things don't fade; they simply find their place within you.

OVERCOMING FEARS

Dr Faatimah Irfaanah Muzammil

Being someone who had just finished her first year in *Paediatrics residency*, my first rotation in my Second year was the *PICU (Paediatric Intensive Care Unit)* rotation. This was my first experience rotating in the PICU. I was filled with fear, anxiety, and excitement. On one hand, I was happy to be able to learn to manage the sickest of patients who were shifted either from the emergency department or from the wards. On the other hand, there was a fear of not exactly knowing my role as a Junior Doctor in the PICU, where the sickest of kids and the most frightened parents and families are.

During the first few days of my PICU rotation, I understood nothing about *sedations* and could not understand most of the *ventilator machines*, which were essential aspects of the intensive department. All I could focus on was how sick the children were, most being intubated and needing medications to maintain their blood pressure and blood supply to their organs. I was fortunate to be with some very knowledgeable and supportive intensive care doctors who were so patient with me, teaching me the basics of *physiology* and explaining how delicate the patient care can be in the ICU.

As time went by, and I had rotated in the PICU more often, I enjoyed the science of medical diseases and felt a sense of fulfilment in being part of the team, which was doing many things to save the children when their condition would suddenly deteriorate.

It was very humbling to see how, even in the cases of acute deterioration and at times of *resuscitation* during *cardiac arrest*, how calm and composed the intensive care doctors were. The idea was to maintain a clear line of thinking, avoid panic, and take the right steps at the right time to save the life of the child. This is because in such situations, every passing second is precious, and every step we take is a deciding moment in the life of the child.

Seeing patients who were almost slipping away from life being revived, then shifted to the wards in a much more stable state, to eventually recover so well that they can be sent home, truly feels like a miracle.

This makes me realise every time that Almighty God has blessed us with the opportunity to serve as doctors, to save lives, and make a difference in the lives of so many families.

In my opinion, every doctor is extremely important, irrespective of their specialty and location of practice, because he/she is making a big difference in the lives of patients and their families.

I am deeply grateful to the Almighty, our parents, and senior doctors for guiding us, young trainees, to overcome fears and grow into confident caregivers.

STEPPING STONES

Anonymous

When I first started medical school, I thought the path to becoming a doctor was going to be a straight line: classes, exams, then on to the hospital. But the reality was far from that. It was full of ups and downs, moments of doubt, and lessons I'll carry with me forever.

In the beginning, I remember feeling overwhelmed by how much information there was to learn. It seemed like I was drowning in textbooks, lectures, and notes every day. At first, I thought the key was to just study more, read and memorise everything. But I quickly learned that this wasn't enough.

One of the biggest turning points for me was realising how important it is to actively engage with the material. It wasn't enough to read; I had to start making diagrams, writing summaries in my own words, and teaching my friends. The more I explained things to others, the more I understood them myself. But even when I felt I was doing everything right, things didn't always go smoothly. During my *internship*, I was thrown into real-world situations, and sometimes, I felt completely unprepared. There's nothing like standing next to a patient who is seriously ill and realising you don't have all the answers.

I had this one experience where a patient's condition suddenly worsened, and I just froze. I was panicking inside, desperately trying to recall everything I'd learned. That moment was humbling. I realised I needed to take a step back, breathe, and focus on what was in front of me. It wasn't about remembering everything perfectly; it was about staying calm and thinking through the problem. That lesson, that it's okay not to have all the answers, was huge for me.

As I moved into *residency*, things got even tougher. The hours were long, and the emotional toll was heavier than I ever expected. I found myself exhausted and burnt out, unsure of how to keep going. It was during this time that I learned one of the most important lessons of all: taking care of myself is just as important as taking care of my patients. I had to get better at managing stress, saying "no" when I needed to, and getting enough sleep.

Looking back, I realise that the hard moments, where I doubted myself or struggled, were the times I learned the most. They shaped me into the doctor I am today. I think what really makes the difference is how you handle the tough times, not just the good ones. And in medicine, those struggles aren't just a part of the process. They're essential in order that we may become compassionate, effective doctors.

If I could offer one piece of advice to future students, it would be this: Don't be afraid to struggle. Lean into those moments. You'll learn so much from them, and they'll help you grow in ways you can't even imagine. The hard times will pass. And when they do, you'll look back and realise that they taught you the lessons that matter most. In the end, it's those lessons you learn through failure, frustration, and perseverance that will not only help you become a better doctor but also make you someone who can truly make a difference in people's lives.

FROM FEARFUL TO FEARLESS

Dr Shabana Muzammil

This story began in the busy streets of a city filled with hustle and life. It started with the admission of an eighteen-year-old into a new world that became accessible after numerous efforts of competitive exams, selections, and interviews.

I was overjoyed and immensely grateful to the Almighty for the final allotment of my medical seat in a small place in Karnataka, 80 km from Bangalore, where I resided in my cosy home. It was 8th August 1990 when we were admitted as a batch of one hundred and fifty students from all over India. As we all entered the college campus, we felt a sense of excitement in working towards attaining the title of 'Doctor.' We were in a room filled with new faces speaking diverse languages.

As we saw the *Anatomy* lab lecture in our schedule, our feet moved with restless joy. Little did we know what the Anatomy lab truly meant. We walked in with pride and enthusiasm, and stumbled in our steps. Shock gripped us as we entered the room that held ten *cadavers* on display, with the smell of *formalin* reeking through them.

We were asked to assemble in groups of fifteen around each dissection table. Although the temperature outside was pleasant and the room was chilly, to our surprise, we could see sweat on each other's faces, especially on our foreheads. As the lecturer started talking, two students fainted. One of the lecturers came running forward to attend to them, and we were told not to get distracted and start the class. We were placed in pairs for every hour, where we had to start the dissection using Cunningham's

Manual. Shivers ran down our spines as my teammate, Satish, and I were called to stand on either side of the palm of the cadaver. With trembling hands, we started our dissection with Kumar Sir's sharp gaze on us. He smiled encouragingly as we made our first incision. We continued learning about different layers and muscle groups, different organs and structures. The days passed into weeks, months and years, and we continued to learn throughout.

It was during this phase that we made friends and grew together. Completing journals while laughing at silly jokes defined some of our fondest memories of that time. Nothing felt more festive than the joy of passing our exams. We were both the guests and the hosts of our celebrations.

As time passed and flew by, we reached *clinicals*, the final years of our training. The dissection and Anatomy lessons we learned transformed into actual cases. The journals we completed became history writing and updating patient files. Amidst all this work and learning, whenever we saw patients with significant exam findings, we used to run to tell our friends to get permission and examine, as this would not only help them in their exams but also in becoming better physicians. A special mention goes to our librarian, who would always keep the latest edition textbooks ready for us and provide us with guidebooks to help us prepare efficiently for exams.

As I stand here and look back at the years of my medical college, I am beyond grateful to the Almighty for this opportunity to become a doctor. I am thankful to my family, professors, and friends who contributed to making those years an enjoyable learning experience for me.

Lastly, I would like to say – to me, anatomy is the king of lessons in a doctor's world as it guides every diagnosis and treatment plan. For this, I would like to humbly thank the cadavers that gave us the knowledge of structure, function, and an appreciation for the value of life. And to remind all of us to help save lives, and that we are all human beings, so we must always try to be humane in our approach.

A DREAM REWRITTEN

Dr Fathima Aaliya Anwar

For as long as I can remember, I have harboured a singular dream: to become a doctor. It wasn't just a career choice - it was the pinnacle of achievement, a symbol of perseverance and intellect. I envisioned the moment I would hold my degree certificate, the culmination of years of rigorous study and relentless dedication. I imagined standing tall, feeling on top of the world, perhaps even basking in a bit of well-earned arrogance. I imagined my heart swelling with pride, convinced that this achievement would mark the apex of my journey.

However, the reality of that moment proved to be starkly different from my fantasies. When I finally grasped my degree certificate, it wasn't a sensation of triumph that washed over me, but a profound sense of indifference. Instead of feeling elated, I felt a void, a blank space where confidence and joy should have resided. The weight of the certificate in my hands felt heavy, not with pride, but with the weight of uncertainty.

I had spent years envisioning this day as the culmination of my efforts, but when it arrived, I was met with a disconcerting emptiness. It was as if the dreams I had meticulously built were crumbling in front of me. I found myself grappling with a gnawing sense of *impostor syndrome*, the belief that I didn't truly deserve this moment, that I was merely an actor in the grand theatre of medicine. My achievements, once so vivid in my dreams, now seemed elusive and hollow.

I looked around and saw the faces of those who had supported me through my journey - family, friends, and mentors. They beamed with pride, but their joy felt like a distant echo compared to the storm of self-doubt raging within me. I felt disconnected from the very dream I had so ardently pursued. The sense of accomplishment that I had envisioned as a grand finale was instead a whisper, overshadowed by confusion and self-doubt.

At that moment, I realised that the journey to becoming a doctor was not merely about acquiring a degree. It was about navigating through a labyrinth of experiences, learning to confront my insecurities, and discovering that the essence of achievement lies not in the certificate, but in the process of becoming. The impostor syndrome I faced was a reminder that the path to self-confidence is fraught with challenges, and that true confidence is a journey, not a destination.

As I stand at the threshold of this new chapter, I understand that the feelings I experienced were not failures, but rather a natural part of the transition from aspiration to reality. My journey has only just begun, and with it comes the realisation that my worth and confidence will not be defined by a certificate alone, but by the continuous pursuit of knowledge, compassion, and self-confidence.

In embracing this, I am learning to rewrite my story - not as a tale of fleeting triumph, but as a journey of growth, resilience, and discovery.

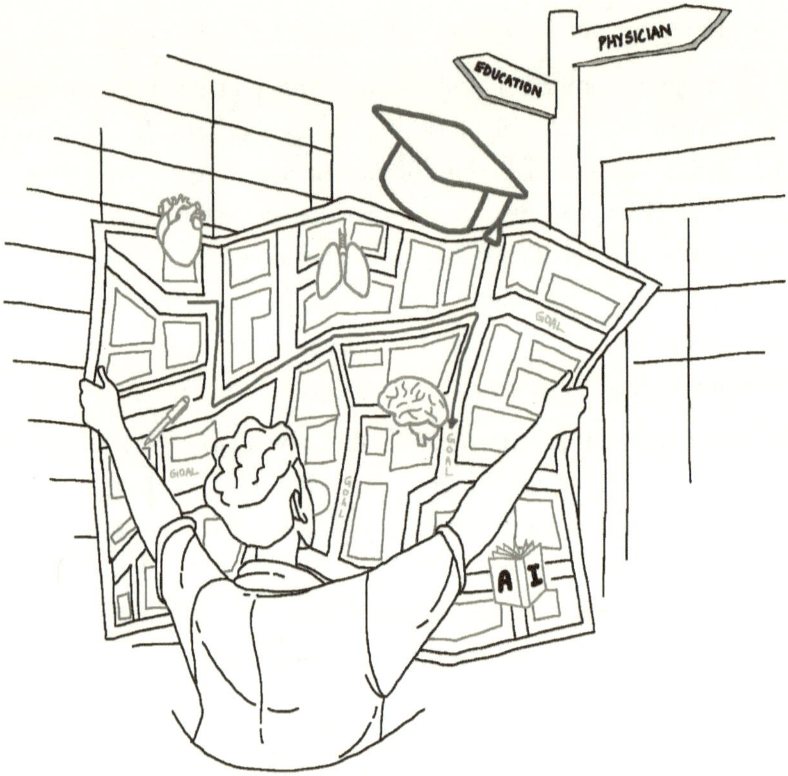

PURPOSE AND PATHWAYS

VEINS OF GRATITUDE

Dr Hana Abdul Kareem

I have always cherished the pursuit of knowledge, but not the kind limited to mere memorisation and cramming, as it is often practised in most places. Instead, I found joy in discovering new words, immersing myself in reading, exploring various subjects, and contemplating the awe-inspiring creations of the Almighty. To be completely honest, during my first year of college, I didn't pay much attention to my lectures. Many times, I found myself sitting there, pondering why I had made this choice in the first place. It was just raining on my parade. But I had to weather the storm.

The *Anatomy* dissection hall was the only place I truly enjoyed returning to. Despite its hideousness and the smell of *formalin*, the atmosphere there sparked my interest. Every time I encountered the *cadavers*, they served as a silent reminder of life's finality, the inevitable reality of death. Strangely, I found comfort in this stark realisation, knowing that whatever challenges I faced were fleeting, much like life in this ephemeral world. Death, the ultimate truth, offered a perspective that brought solace amid life's struggles.

Upon seeing the wide variety of specimens and bones displayed in the hall, my mind was drawn to ponder the intricacies of the human body – its functions, quirks, and enduring mysteries. I couldn't help but marvel at the Exalted for His miraculous creations. It was during one of our sleepy afternoon sessions that our Anatomy professor mentioned the jugular veins. Jugular veins are key players in the circulation and drainage systems to the brain, face, and neck. Most importantly, they drain the brain. If you block the jugular veins, the pressure in the brain goes up."

It hit me like a comet. Jugular vein. It reminded me of a verse in the *Holy Qur'an*. "And We have already created man and know what his soul whispers to him, and We are closer to him than [his] jugular vein." (50:16) It took time for me to realise that, in my negligence, I was missing out on something far greater. I had to embrace gratitude for the path I've been given - the chance to learn, to ponder, to reflect, and to contribute something of value to the world.

And so, I whispered a prayer, "May the Almighty help us learn and serve for His sake, and help us appreciate His creations always and in all ways."

BALANCING THE SCALPEL AND MOTHERHOOD

Dr Sheeba Mariyam

My journey to becoming a surgeon was fuelled by a deep-seated passion ignited in my childhood. From as far back as I can remember, I was fascinated by the intricate human body. As I progressed through school, my interest in science and medicine only grew. When it came time to choose a career path, I had no doubt in my mind - I wanted to be a doctor. Later, more specifically, I wanted to be a surgeon.

I enrolled in medical school, where my curiosity and determination were further fuelled by the complexities of human anatomy and the challenges of patient care. Each lecture and practical session solidified my resolve. I vividly remember my first experience in the operating room. The atmosphere was intense, the stakes high, and every movement precise. The surgeon, calm and focused, worked methodically, explaining every little cut he made and why. Watching the procedure, I felt an overwhelming sense of purpose. I knew for sure at that moment that surgery was where I belonged.

Surgery combined everything I loved about medicine: the ability to make an immediate, tangible difference, the challenge of complex problem-solving, and the opportunity to work with my hands in a precise and skilled manner. I saw surgery as an art form, each procedure a masterpiece crafted with knowledge, skill, and care.

The road to becoming a surgeon was demanding. Long hours of study, gruelling shifts, and the constant pressure to excel were part of the job. There were moments of doubt and exhaustion, but my passion never wavered. I was driven by the calling of countless patients who needed someone to take decisive action to save their lives.

As I progressed through my *residency*, I faced an additional challenge: balancing my career with motherhood. Being a mother of two young children added a layer of complexity to an already demanding profession. Early mornings, late nights, and unpredictable hours became the norm. There were moments when the guilt of not being able to spend more time with my children weighed heavily on me. I had to constantly juggle between the demands of my patients and the needs of my family.

The support of my spouse and family was crucial during this time. They understood my passion and helped create a nurturing environment for our children. Despite the challenges, I found strength in knowing that I was setting an example for my children, demonstrating the importance of pursuing one's passion and the value of hard work and dedication.

Throughout my residency, I honed my skills and learned from experienced surgeons who became my mentors. They taught me not only the technical aspects of surgery but also the importance of empathy, patience, and precision. I learned that being a surgeon was not just about performing procedures, but about caring for patients, understanding their fears, and guiding them through some of the most challenging times of their lives.

Now, as a practising surgeon, I carry those lessons with me every day. Each patient I meet, each surgery I perform, is a reminder of why I chose this path. It is a privilege to be able to heal, to restore, and to give hope. Becoming a surgeon was not just a career choice; it was a calling, a passion that continues to drive me, inspire me, and define who I am.

Balancing the roles of a surgeon and a mother is a continuous challenge, but it is one that I embrace wholeheartedly. In every surgery, I strive to honour the trust my patients place in me. Their courage and strength motivate me to give my best, to keep learning, and to keep improving. And with each life I touch, I am reminded of the profound impact that one person's passion can have on the world.

FROM HEALING HANDS TO SHAPING MINDS

Dr Fouzia Shersad V

I still recall the thrill of clinic days - soaking in grateful smiles, diving into spirited academic debates, and offering a healing touch to calm anxious hearts. I never imagined stepping out without my medical kit or considering a different professional identity. Although I was thankful for the warm praise from patients and colleagues who recognised my dedication and empathy, I felt the gentle pull of family commitments nudging me like a breeze. My children were blossoming each day, and I wanted to be present in their ever-evolving world. With my *nephrologist* husband perpetually *on-call*, I longed for more time together. Believing a "nine-to-five" might bring balance, I took a leap - unaware that this new path would consume even more hours, yet spark a passion and excitement beyond anything I had imagined.

When I arrived in Dubai in 2001, I had a strong intuition that guided me towards academia. Although leaving full-time clinical work felt daunting, I soon discovered how fulfilling it is to teach future physicians. Educating students multiplied my contribution to patient care exponentially; a single lesson could affect countless lives through the doctors I helped train. My clinical background turned out to be a remarkable asset in the classroom - right from day one, I was able to guide medical students on the realities of patient interactions and genuine human suffering.

I found my stride in teaching *pathology*, which sits at the intersection of basic science and clinical practice. This vantage point allowed me to connect theoretical concepts with real-world patient outcomes, bridging the gap for students between what they learn in lectures and what they observe in hospitals. My growing fascination with assessment as a driving force in student learning, along with my interest in quality management, led me to discover an exciting new focus within medical education - one that bridged the clinical setting with the educational journey leading up to it.

A successful interview at Dubai Medical College (DMC) soon became a turning point, placing me in roles that ranged from Associate Professor to Director of Medical Education and Quality over the next two decades. Working alongside a dedicated team, we navigated rigorous accreditation processes and eventually celebrated the status as the only educational institution in Dubai to receive the prestigious Dubai Quality Award (DQA). It was a shared moment of pride for everyone involved when we earned the Mohammed Bin Rashid Al Maktoum (MRM) Award and the World Education Congress Awards in 2011.

Paradoxically, my supposed move to "less demanding" academic work placed me at the forefront of new challenges that devoured my time and attention, but it was exhilarating. Fuelled by my clinical expertise, I took on the task of shaping medical curricula, focusing on professionalism and quality assurance, which eventually inspired me to pursue a PhD concentrating on quality management in medical education. My FAIMER project revolved around professionalism as well, reinforcing my conviction that empathy, ethics, and communication are as vital as scientific knowledge in producing well-rounded physicians.

Once I delved into the finer points of quality management, I began to see education as a living ecosystem, much like the human body, where every part needs nurturing for the whole to flourish. Embracing this expanded outlook, I stepped into a role as a Senior Assessor for the Dubai Quality Award, which nudged me beyond the lecture hall and deepened my resolve to raise standards wherever learning takes place. Along the way, I found myself organising international conferences, shaping competency frameworks, and sparking new ideas on how to better equip the next generation of doctors. Still, the most memorable moments were those devoted to social initiatives and initiating summer electives, where students got a real taste of patient care and service to the community.

When I look back, my clinical background gave me a special vantage point. Every experience with patients helped me show students and colleagues how the theories in textbooks come alive in busy hospital corridors. I also learned firsthand that juggling family and professional goals can be done with flexibility and a supportive network, even if it means following a winding path instead of a neat "nine-to-five."

Today, I carry this perspective into my work as a Medical Education Expert at the National Institute for Health Specialities (NIHS) in the UAE, where I collaborate with teams to shape Emirati Board exams and workplace-based assessments. I consider it a privilege to guide postgraduate training, setting the stage for excellence through national board examinations. I also lend my insights to global medical education initiatives as a Project Adviser at the International FAIMER Institute in Philadelphia. My enthusiasm for lifelong learning, continuous professional development (CPD), and new frontiers like integrating Artificial Intelligence (AI) into assessments keeps me immersed in research and innovation. Each new venture reminds me that education, much like a blossoming garden, thrives on vision, empathy, and the flexibility to grow alongside those who nurture it.

As I look back on my thirty-year trajectory from comforting patients at the bedside to academic leadership, I have realised that there is no single path in medicine that outshines another. While direct patient care offered immediate rewards, training the next generation of physicians has multiplied that sense of purpose a hundredfold. My clinical insight became the bridge that led students towards deeper empathy and professional excellence. This journey has taught me that while healing lives is noble, shaping minds can create a ripple effect that extends far beyond a single patient. It is a legacy I am proud to leave behind.

FROM TEST TUBES TO TENNIS COURTS

Dr Tanaz George

During my medical school days, amidst the rigorous hours of studying and intense exams, the *biochemistry* and *physiology* labs were where our paths first crossed. It was there that I met George, a fellow student with a passion for tennis that matched his dedication to medicine. Our roll numbers were next to each other, which meant we often ended up being lab partners.

The labs were places of intense focus, with students meticulously studying *metabolic pathways*, *enzyme* functions, and the complexities of human physiology. On the first day of our biochemistry course, I found myself assigned to a group that included George. He stood out immediately - tall, athletic, and with a calm demeanour that contrasted with the usual nerves of first-year medical students.

Over the weeks, our group worked closely together, and I quickly noticed that George was incredibly kind, always ready to help others in our group. Outside the lab, I discovered that George was an avid tennis player. He often talked about his matches and how tennis helped him manage the stress of medical school. One afternoon, after a particularly challenging physiology lab, George invited me to watch one of his tennis matches. Intrigued, I agreed. Watching George on the tennis court was a revelation. It was clear that the discipline and focus he applied in the lab were mirrored on the court.

During one of our clinical rounds, our Head of Department (HoD) discussed a complex case on *brain tumour*. We stood nervously as the HoD fired challenging questions about the case. The case was so challenging that even the postgraduate students struggled to answer. A while ago, George had discussed the very case with his dad, a seasoned doctor, over dinner. His father, Dr Varghese, had shared a critical insight that tied together seemingly unrelated symptoms and pointed to a rare but treatable condition. Drawing on that conversation, George took a deep breath and confidently addressed the HoD's question, outlining the diagnostic approach and treatment plan his father had suggested. George's ability to integrate his father's wisdom into his professional expertise was truly admirable.

Eventually, our medical school journey culminated in not just attaining the degree, but also in a beautiful wedding with the presence of our family and friends.

Beyond medical school, I chose to specialise in *pathology*, fascinated by the intricacies of disease processes and diagnostics. George, on the other hand, pursued *orthopaedics*, combining his love for sports with his medical career. He eventually established himself in *sports medicine*, helping athletes recover from injuries and optimise their performance. He had combined both his passions and pursued a holistic pathway, reminding us that to practise medicine, one doesn't have to sacrifice hobbies and interests. Instead, we can integrate them together, allowing us to pursue them both on a unique path with a profound purpose.

Looking back, even after two decades, George and I often reminisce about those early days, grateful for the serendipity of roll numbers that led us to each other. Our careers have taken different paths, but our commitment to each other and our shared journey in medicine have always kept us connected.

MY PATH TO BLENDING MEDICINE WITH ARTIFICIAL INTELLIGENCE

Dr Shifan Khanday

My journey into the world of medicine began not just with an aspiration to heal, but with a profound desire to understand the human body in all its intricate complexities. The first steps were taken at Jammu, India, where I pursued my MBBS. Those years were transformative, deepening my passion for *anatomy* and fuelling my quest for medical knowledge.

Yet, the path was strewn with obstacles. Early in my career, I faced a pivotal moment when I had to forgo pursuing surgery due to differing career paths between my spouse and me. This detour, though initially felt as a setback, steered me towards the realms of basic medical sciences and education, and a reacquaintance with family medicine. This wasn't just a shift in my career trajectory; it was an expansion of my perspective, allowing me to embrace the multidimensional nature of medicine.

Driven by relentless curiosity, I sought further education globally – from a Doctorate in *Anatomy* to a Diploma in Family Medicine from RCGP, London, a Master's in Health Professions Education, an MBA in Healthcare, and a PhD specialising in anatomical variations. This a fifteen-plus-year academic journey was a testament to my commitment to understanding every detail of human anatomy.

A significant turning point in my career was the integration of Artificial Intelligence (AI) into healthcare. AI offered a promising new frontier, enhancing diagnostic accuracy, personalising patient care, and ultimately revolutionising traditional medical practices.

My venture into AI was driven not just by professional ambition but by the necessity to stay at the forefront of medical innovation. I pursued an MSc in Artificial Intelligence in Healthcare in Spain, which equipped me to lead in this transformative field.

Acknowledging the critical role of AI in the future of medicine, I championed the integration of an AI course into the curriculum at Dubai Medical University. This initiative was designed to prepare medical students for a future where technology and healthcare converge, equipping them with the skills to use AI tools both effectively and ethically.

In ensuring the responsible application of AI, I played a key role in drafting an ethical use policy for AI at our institution. This policy serves as a foundational guide for both students and professionals, helping them navigate the ethical complexities they may encounter when using AI in medical settings.

My commitment to expanding knowledge on the potential and challenges of AI in healthcare also led me to author the book, "AI and I: Basics of Artificial Intelligence in Healthcare and Medical Education." This publication bridges the gap between complex AI technologies and their practical applications in healthcare.

Furthermore, recognising the necessity for a platform to nurture and accelerate innovative AI solutions in healthcare, I established an accelerator programme. This initiative promotes collaboration among technologists, healthcare professionals, and academics, facilitating the rapid development and implementation of AI technologies that can reshape patient care and healthcare management.

Now, as I lead the AI and Smart Education Unit at Dubai Medical University, I am focused on weaving AI into every aspect of medical education and practice. Our projects range from

AI-driven diagnostic tools to intelligent learning platforms, all designed to prepare future medical professionals for a new era in healthcare.

The emotional essence of my journey into AI has been fuelled by a dedication to using technology to enhance compassionate care. The road has been fraught with challenges - overcoming scepticism, bridging the divide between technology and patient care, and continuously adapting to rapid technological advancements. Each challenge has strengthened my determination to blend my medical expertise with AI, aiming to improve educational methodologies and enhance diagnostic and therapeutic outcomes.

This story, my story, is not just about observing the evolution of medicine, but actively driving it. Standing on the threshold of the next medical revolution, my journey from a medical student to an AI expert encapsulates an unending quest for knowledge, betterment, and, most importantly, the relentless pursuit of enhancing human lives.

MORE ABOUT THE AUTHORS

Dr Ahila Abu-Nayla *is currently an Anaesthesia and Critical Care Resident at American Hospital Dubai. Inspired by her father, a dedicated physician, she developed a deep interest in medicine from an early age. She graduated from Dubai Medical University in 2023 and remains driven by a commitment to advancing healthcare and delivering compassionate patient care. Her rigorous training in anaesthesia and critical care has equipped her with expertise in managing high-acuity cases and perioperative medicine. Outside clinical duties, she contributes to medical education through workshops and case presentations, fostering a culture of knowledge-sharing. She is particularly passionate about optimising pain management protocols and improving outcomes for critically ill patients.*

Dr Aiman Hidayat *is a dedicated medical intern at Khyber Teaching Hospital. Born and raised in the UAE, she pursued her MBBS in Pakistan, driven by a passion for serving humanity. Aiman aims to specialise in Obstetrics and Gynaecology, providing compassionate care to women in underserved communities. Outside of medicine, she enjoys painting, travelling, reading fiction, and organising events. As an Overseas Student Ambassador at Shaukat Khanum Memorial Cancer Hospital and a public speaker at awareness events organised by her college, she has demonstrated exceptional leadership and communication skills. She aspires to become a skilled gynaecologist, making a meaningful difference in the lives of those in need, particularly the poor and vulnerable.*

Dr Anaam Parveen *is a medical graduate passionate about medicine and neuroscience, aspiring to blend her love for storytelling with her dedication to helping others. She believes in the power of words to inspire growth and foster understanding, using her unique perspective to explore the intricate connections between health, the mind, and human experience. She is working on her first book, where she aims to share insights from her journey in medicine, weaving together personal stories and scientific knowledge to empower readers.*

When she finds time off from studying, she enjoys crocheting, reading, crafts, and writing, and is excited to connect with fellow writers and readers on this journey.

Dr Aya Mohammed Ali Alsabbah *is currently an intern at the Mohammed Bin Rashid University of Medicine and Health Sciences (MBRU). She graduated from Dubai Medical College with a Bachelor's degree in Medicine and Surgery. Her journey through medical school and her ongoing internship have been deeply enriching, offering insights that go far beyond the technical aspects of medicine. She is especially passionate about the power of small, thoughtful actions in improving patient care. As she continues her professional path, she is dedicated to refining her clinical skills and discovering where she can make the most meaningful impact.*

Dr Faatimah Maryam Muzammil *is a passionate individual who believes that medicine is an art and a science. She aims to create a community where quality healthcare is accessible to all those who need it. She is an advocate for physical and mental health for the people around her. She is an active volunteer in healthcare and non-healthcare-related fields. She has received national and international awards for her work in different fields. Outside of work, she loves spending time on her hobbies of reading, creativity, and fun, along with her family and friends.*

Dr Faatimah Irfaanah Muzammil *is a paediatrician and a strong believer that the idea of health and well-being should be promoted in individuals right from their childhood so that they have healthy habits from a young age. She is an advocate for promoting good parent-child relations, as it has a significant impact on the physical, mental, and emotional well-being of children as they enter adulthood. As an active campaigner for health and wellness, she has won the International Diana Award from the UK, among many other national and international laurels. She also enjoys artwork, creative work, and reading storybooks.*

Dr Hana Abdul Kareem *is a dedicated intern with a lifelong passion for writing. Originally from Kannur, Kerala, she completed her schooling in*

Al Ain, UAE. She enjoys playing with words to weave hope and express a range of emotions, using her craft to help herself and others navigate life's challenges while reminding everyone of its ultimate purpose. She recently authored a poetry collection titled "Poesy," which is currently available on various online platforms. In addition to her poetry, she has contributed to numerous magazines, research works, and anthologies, earning accolades in various writing, public speaking, and quiz competitions, including several prestigious contests.

Hurairah Faatimah Muzammil *is an accomplished and passionate member of the medical field, recognised for her exceptional contributions to healthcare, public service, and global advocacy. She has been a recipient of prestigious international, national and regional awards. Beyond medicine, she is a passionate public speaker and dedicated volunteer, actively participating in health campaigns, awareness programmes, and sustainability initiatives. Her leadership has shone on international platforms, including roles as a panellist at events like COP28 and COY18, where they championed global health and environmental causes. Through a commitment to research, education, and community service, she continues to inspire positive change on both local and international levels.*

Dr Lekshmi Nath *earned her MBBS from Government Medical College, Kottayam, which she followed up with DGO from Calicut Medical College and then DNB (Obstetrics and Gynaecology). She started her career as a lecturer and is currently serving as a professor. She has also completed special training in Laparoscopy and Infertility treatment.*

Dr Mariyam Thahira *is currently a medical intern, who aspires to pursue further clinical training, alongside contributing to medical research, healthcare accessibility, and quality. She graduated from Dubai Medical College. Previously, she published a poetry compilation titled 'Earthen Po(e)t-ry' and was Chief Editor and Co-head of design for the college magazine, as well as Co-founder of DMC Quran Programme.*

Dr Marwa Abdelmagid *from Khartoum, Sudan, is currently an intern in the UAE. With a spirit of resilience, she graduated with distinction during a time of war in her home country, demonstrating remarkable strength and determination. Beyond her professional pursuits, she embraces her adventurous side through horse riding and ice skating, balancing her ambitions with her passions. Guided by a philosophy rooted in faith that 'God will always choose and give what's best for us, even if we didn't see it,' she continually strives for excellence, never settling for anything less than the stars.*

Dr Meharish Ambatt *is a general surgeon based in Dubai with roots in Kerala, India. Even before her medical school days, she knew surgery was her path, and in her own words, 'went to medicine to come out as a surgeon, not just as a doctor.' Driven by this goal, she pursued a General Surgery residency in Dubai and became the first Indian medical graduate to be accepted into the programme. She believes that luck is when preparation meets opportunity, and consistent hard work always bears fruit. Currently navigating life as a new mother, she continues her journey as a surgeon practising in Dubai and runs a platform to guide aspiring doctors on residency pathways and share motivation within the medical community. She hopes to inspire future surgeons, especially female surgeons, to chase after their dreams unapologetically and to lead by example.*

Dr Mohammed Shaamin *is a curious soul disguised as a doctor. A South Indian by roots and a dreamer by default, he juggles postgraduate entrance exam preparation, research aspirations, and the occasional food truck fantasy. When he's not buried in medical videos, he's probably sketching out a new outfit idea, reading about ancient civilisations, or plotting ways to make science a little more human. He believes in thoughtful work, good coffee, and changing the world, one life at a time.*

Dr Muzammil Hafeez *is a neonatologist by profession and an outstanding one at that. With over twenty-five years of experience, he is a Member of the Royal College of Paediatrics and Child Health and has attained degrees and a fellowship in the field. He is passionate about healthcare, research,* *and teaching as he believes, "We rise by lifting others."* He *is keen about participating in walks, camps, awareness campaigns, and much more for social causes and healthcare services. With a zest for knowledge and good work, he continues to inspire and train the next generation of competent residents and remarkable doctors.*

Dr Rawan Ahmed Mehanna *is a clinical faculty member in the Clinical Sciences department at Dubai Medical University and a keen Simulation Educator. With a passion for neurology, she combines her expertise with a love for gamification and simulation in medical education. Through her writing, she delves into the transformative experiences and lessons learned throughout her medical journey. Her contribution to this book stems from a desire to share the complexities, challenges, and rewards of being a doctor, offering insights and inspiration to fellow young medical professionals and readers alike.*

Dr Riya Azeez *is a 2019 MBBS graduate from Amrita Institute of Medical Sciences, Kochi. She currently works as a General Duty Medical Officer at Meitra Hospital in Calicut, India. Born and raised in Dubai, she completed her schooling at GEMS Our Own English High School. Dr Riya aspires to pursue postgraduate studies in Internal Medicine or an allied field. In her free time, she enjoys reading, learning new languages, and gardening. Through her journey in medicine, she has come to value the humbling truth that there is always something new to learn each day, a perspective she hopes to share with readers through her writing.*

Rushda Haider *is an undergraduate medical student at Dubai Medical University, with a strong passion for surgery and anaesthesiology. Known for her dynamic leadership and ability to balance academics with extracurriculars, she currently holds several roles: Secretary of the Volunteering Committee, Treasurer of the Student Council, Preclinical Representative of the Surgical Club, Local Committee Representative for IFMSA-UAE, and Co-Outreach Coordinator for IASSS UAE. Rushda has also contributed to numerous national and international events, workshops, and research projects, including* *a published mini-review. Her commitment to community engagement and medical education continues to drive her towards her goal of becoming an impactful healthcare professional.*

Dr Salam Chettian Kandi, *MBBS; MS (Ophthalmology), is an ophthalmologist with over twenty-five years of experience in clinical and surgical eye care, currently serving at Hospitals under Dubai Health, UAE. He is especially skilled in anterior segment surgeries and other ophthalmic procedures. He graduated from Kasturba Medical College, Mangalore, India (1997), with a commitment to evidence-based, compassionate care. He is also passionate about improving access to eye health services in underserved communities and mentoring the next generation of healthcare professionals.*

Dr Shameema Alam *graduated from Dubai Medical University, UAE. As a co-author of "Beats of their Drums," she is also a published poet. The hobbies she enjoys most are writing English and Urdu poetry and volunteering. She is also a registered volunteer in the UAE government's volunteering programme and is passionate about volunteering for social causes. She is an active participant in many of her college clubs that involve volunteering, poetry, writing and medical skills. At her college, she was the former Head of the Scientific Committee, and she organised a lot of scientific events to spread awareness about different health conditions inside and outside the college. Furthermore, she organised book-related events at college as the former head of the book club.*

Dr Shabana Muzammil *is a dedicated physician with a passion for creating positive societal impact. She holds an MBBS, a Master's in Health Sciences (Diabetes), and a Fellowship in Diabetology from the UK, along with a Level-7 Diploma in Strategic Management and Leadership. With over twenty years of teaching experience, she has educated students from diverse backgrounds, empowering them with knowledge and growth opportunities. She has contributed to national and international health campaigns, driven by her vision for global change. A natural leader and team player, she combines strategic thinking with compassion, inspiring the next generation of doctors* *through academics and mentorship. She believes every individual effort counts toward global progress. Her life motto: Do what you love and love what you do.*

Dr Sheeba Mariyam V K *is a General and Laparoscopic Surgeon currently serving in the Sultanate of Oman. She is known for her expertise in minimally invasive procedures, compassionate patient care, and dedication to surgical education. A graduate of MES Medical College with a Master's in General Surgery from Azeezia Medical College, India, she was actively involved in mentoring medical students and trainees in Malabar Medical College until she moved to Oman. Dr Sheeba combines clinical precision with academic engagement and is passionate about fostering a culture of excellence in healthcare.*

Dr Shyam Kishan *is a Paediatric Orthopaedic and Spine Surgeon, an American Board-certified orthopaedic surgeon with over thirty years of experience, specialising in Paediatric spinal deformities and complex musculoskeletal conditions. A proud graduate of JIPMER, India, Dr Kishan completed advanced training in the U.S, including a Paediatric orthopaedic fellowship at Rady Children's Hospital, San Diego. Currently serving as Medical Director of Paediatric Orthopaedics & Trauma at Medical City Children's Hospital, Dallas, and faculty at the Southwest Scoliosis and Spine Institute. He is recognised for his work in scoliosis correction (growing rods, Mehta casting, vertebral body tethering), limb deformity, hip dysplasia, and neuromuscular conditions like cerebral palsy and spina bifida. He also helps take care of children with spinal deformities in Mexico twice every year as part of the Global Spine Outreach organisation's mission. Passionate about compassionate care, cutting-edge techniques, and mentoring future surgeons.*

Dr Srutdi Kamalam Natarajan *is a dedicated physician from India who also has a great passion for music, art, and creative writing. She is dedicated to quality patient care, innovative research, and community health initiatives. She loves collaborating with like-minded people and seeking new avenues for creative exploration. Through her experiences as a medical student, she wishes to illuminate the various facets of the profession - the positive,* *negative, and challenging aspects. She appreciates a good sense of humour, so much so that her favourite bone in the body is the humerus.*

Dr Suhaila Ahmed *is a dedicated medical intern at Mohammed Bin Rashid University of Medicine and Health Sciences (MBRU), Dubai Health, with a focus on General Surgery. A 2024 honours graduate of Dubai Medical College for Girls and an upcoming General Surgery Resident, she combines hands-on clinical experience with compassionate patient care. As a former batch leader and National Delegate at IASSS UAE, Suhaila has led initiatives bridging medical education and community service. Beyond medicine, she enjoys writing poetry, singing, and mentoring future healthcare professionals. She aspires to become a surgeon, academic, and advocate for holistic, patient-centred care.*

Dr Sumaiyya Shersad *is a dedicated NHS Family Physician based at Longton Hall Surgery in Stoke-on-Trent. With a strong foundation in general practice, she provides comprehensive, patient-centred care focused on preventive health, chronic disease management, and family well-being. Known for her empathetic approach and clinical diligence, she is committed to improving lives across the community she serves.*

Dr Tasnim Mustafa *graduated from Dubai Medical University with a deep interest in Paediatrics and dermatology. She is currently involved in a research project exploring the relationship between the severity of acne vulgaris and vitamin D levels, aiming to contribute to the growing body of evidence in dermatological health. She is passionate about integrating clinical practice with research to enhance patient care and outcomes. Her long-term goal is to empower individuals, especially young patients, by helping them feel confident in their skin and overall health through compassionate care, education, and evidence-based medical approaches.*

Dr Tasnima Tayb *is an intern who undertakes ambitious projects towards humanitarian betterment, research excellence, and public health. Through campaigning for blood donation awareness, youth leadership, and educational awareness, she is a resilient visionary and action-taker who* *champions community welfare. Curious, determined, and driven, her other passions include spoken word poetry, debate, and graphic design.*

Dr Vinidh Paleri *is a Consultant Head and Neck Surgeon at The Royal Marsden NHS Foundation Trust, London. Specialising in complex cancer surgeries, he is dedicated to advancing patient care through precision medicine and compassionate treatment. He featured prominently in Channel Four's documentary series one and two, Super Surgeons: A Chance at Life, which offers a rare glimpse into the realities of modern surgical oncology. Beyond the operating theatre, he is passionate about medical education, research and sharing stories that highlight the human side of healthcare.*

LinkedIn

- Amna Ibrahim Zaidan
- Anaam Parveen
- Aisha Ismail Makandar
- Aya Alsabbah
- Asra'a Alnakeb
- Fouzia Shersad
- Dr. Fathima Aaliya Anwar
- Maryam Rahmatullah
- Maya Elmaghraby
- Dr.Meharish Ambatt
- Noor Mohamed
- Raabeah Fatma Jafri
- Dr. Rawan Mehanna
- Salam Chettiankandi
- Shaista Khadim MBBS
- Shameema Alam
- Shifan Khanday
- Dr. Sheeba Mariyam
- Srutdi Kamalam Natarajan
- Sobia Mir
- Tiba Aldelaimi
- Vinidh Paleri

GLOSSARY

A

Abscess - A collection of pus that forms due to infection, often causing pain, swelling etc.

Adenosine - A medication used to quickly restore normal heart rhythm in certain types of fast, irregular heartbeats.

Adrenaline - A hormone that the body releases in stressful or emergency situations. Doctors also use it in emergencies, such as severe allergic reactions or cardiac arrest, among others.

Alternating Hemiplegia of Childhood - A rare condition in young children where one side of the body suddenly becomes weak or paralysed, but the episodes go away and switch sides over time.

Anatomy - A study of the structure and parts of the body, like bones, muscles, organs, etc.

Anaemia - A condition where there aren't enough healthy red blood cells in the body, making one feel tired, weak, or short of breath.

Anaesthesia - Medicines used during surgeries to block pain, either creating numbness in one area or putting you completely to sleep.

OR, the department specialising in inducing that state for surgery or other procedures.

Anencephaly - A serious birth defect where a baby is born without parts of the brain and skull.

Antenatal – Before the birth of a baby, or, in other words, during pregnancy.

Aortic Stenosis - A heart problem where the main valve (aortic valve) becomes too narrow, making it hard for blood to flow out of the heart.

Appendectomy - A surgery to remove the appendix, usually done when someone has appendicitis (infection of the appendix).

Arthritis - Swelling and pain in the joints, which makes them stiff, painful, and difficult to move.

Attending - A fully trained senior doctor who supervises and guides junior doctors and medical students in the hospital.

Auscultation - Listening to the sounds of the body, usually with a stethoscope, to check the heart, lungs, or intestines.

Axillary - A medical term for the armpit area.

B

Beta Thalassaemia - A blood disorder with a defect in the haemoglobin, which is a component of red blood cells.

Benign - A benign lump or growth that isn't cancerous.

Biochemistry - The study of chemical processes that occur within living organisms, especially related to metabolism and cellular function.

Biopsy - A small sample of tissue taken from the body to look at under a microscope. Doctors use it to check for things like cancer or infection, among others.

Bone Marrow Aspiration - A procedure that involves extracting a small amount of bone marrow, typically from the hip bone, to examine blood cell production.

Brain tumour - An abnormal lump or growth of cells in the brain.

Brainstem reflexes - Body responses controlled by the lower part of the brain. Doctors check these to understand if the brain is still working, especially in very sick or unconscious patients.

C

Cadaver - A dead human body through which medical students and doctors study and learn about the structure and parts of the body.

Cardiac Arrest - It's a medical emergency where the heart suddenly stops beating, causing the person to stop breathing and lose consciousness.

Cardiology - The branch of medicine that deals with the heart and blood vessels.

Cautery - A method doctors use to stop bleeding or remove tissue by burning it with heat or electricity.

Cerebral palsy - A group of conditions caused by brain damage before or after birth that affects movement, balance, and muscle control.

Chemotherapy - Strong medicines used to kill cancer cells.

Chest tube - A flexible tube inserted into the space of the chest between the lungs and the layer of tissue covering it. It is often used to drain air, blood, or fluid and allow the lungs to move freely.

Chief Complaint - The primary symptom or concern that prompts a patient to seek medical attention. It reflects the patient's own words or focus and is not a diagnosis.

Chronic - A long-lasting condition that doesn't go away easily and often needs ongoing care (like diabetes or arthritis).

Cholecystitis - Inflammation (swelling and pain) of the gallbladder, often caused by gallstones.

Cholecystectomy - Surgery to remove the gallbladder.

Clinical phase - The part of medical training where students work with real patients in hospitals to learn hands-on skills.

CPR (Cardiopulmonary Resuscitation) - An emergency procedure that combines chest compressions and breaths to restore circulation and breathing in cardiac arrest.

Crackles/crepitations - Crackling or popping sounds a doctor hears through a stethoscope when listening to the lungs. Often a sign of fluid or infection in the lungs.

Cranial nerve - These are special nerves that come from the brain and control things like seeing, hearing, facial movement, swallowing, etc.

Crepitations - Another word for crackling sounds heard in the lungs, can also mean a crunching sound when bones or joints rub abnormally.

Crowning - During childbirth, it's the moment the baby's head becomes visible.

Code Blue - A hospital emergency alert indicating that the resuscitation team is needed immediately.

Colostomy - A surgery where a part of the large intestine (colon) is brought to the skin surface to pass waste into a bag, often after part of the bowel is removed.

Commode chair - A portable chair with a toilet seat, used by people who have trouble walking to the bathroom.

Comorbidity - When someone has more than one medical condition at the same time, like diabetes and high blood pressure together.

Congenital - A condition or problem that a person is born with, like a heart defect.

Consultant - A highly experienced and senior doctor who leads a medical team and is an expert in a specific field.

D

Defibrillator - A machine that uses an electric shock to the heart to regulate an abnormal heart rhythm.

Dermatology - The branch of medicine that is related to diseases of the skin, hair, nails, and related structures.

Diabetes - A condition where the body can't properly control sugar levels in the blood, either because it doesn't make enough insulin or can't use it well.

Disc Herniation - When a spinal disc's inner material pushes out through a tear in its outer layer, often pressing on nearby nerves.

Discharge Against Medical Advice (DAMA) - When a patient chooses to leave the hospital before the doctor recommends it, even if it might not be safe.

DOCEE (Direct Observation Clinical Encounter Examination) - A type of medical school exam where the student is watched while they care for a real patient, taking history, examining, and making diagnoses.

E

ECG (Electrocardiogram) - A test that records the electrical activity of the heart to check for problems like irregular beats or heart attacks.

Ectopic pregnancy - A pregnancy where the baby starts growing outside the womb, usually in the tube. It's dangerous and needs urgent treatment.

Epicondyle - A bony bump near a joint (like the elbow or knee) where muscles attach.

Epigastric - The upper central part of the abdomen.

ENT / Otorhinolaryngology - The medical specialty that deals with problems of the Ear, Nose, and Throat.

Enzyme - Tiny proteins in the body that help speed up chemical reactions, like breaking down food or helping cells work properly.

ER (Emergency Room) - The hospital department providing immediate treatment for sudden illnesses and injuries that need urgent care.

F

Fallopian tube - A part of the female reproductive system that carries eggs from the ovaries to the womb (uterus); it's where fertilisation usually happens.

Febrile neutropenia - A condition where a person has a fever and very low white blood cells (which fight infection), often seen in cancer patients receiving chemotherapy. It's a medical emergency.

Femoral vein - A large vein in the upper thigh that carries blood from the leg back to the heart.

Femur - The thigh bone, the longest and strongest bone in the human body.

Fibroadenoma - A common, non-cancerous lump in the breast, often found in young women. It usually feels smooth and moves easily under the skin.

Fibroid - A non-cancerous growth in the uterus (womb) that can cause heavy periods, pain or fertility issues.

Formalin - A strong chemical used in labs to preserve body tissues.

Fossa - A shallow dip or hollow in a bone that holds muscles or organs.

Fungating – A mass that grows similar to a fungus in its appearance.

G

Gauze - A soft, thin fabric used to clean wounds or stop bleeding; often placed over cuts or surgical sites.

Gestational – Anything related to pregnancy.

Glioblastoma Multiforme - A highly aggressive and malignant type of brain tumour arising from glial cells, known for its rapid progression and poor prognosis.

Gurney - A hospital stretcher with wheels, used to move patients.

Gynaecomastia - Enlargement of breast tissue in males, usually due to hormonal imbalance or certain medications.

H

Hadith - A religious term that refers to the recorded sayings or actions of the Prophet Muhammad (peace be upon him) as per Islamic teachings.

Heave - A visible lifting of the chest wall that can be seen or felt, often during a heart examination, suggesting the heart is working harder than normal.

Hemothorax - Accumulation of blood in the space between the lungs and chest wall, often due to trauma or injury, among others.

History - In medicine, the detailed account of a patient's symptoms, past illnesses, and lifestyle, gathered during a clinical interview.

Hippocratic Oath - A promise doctors make to treat people ethically and do no harm.

Hypoglycaemia - A condition where blood glucose levels drop below normal, potentially causing symptoms like sweating, confusion and fainting.

Hypertension - High blood pressure, a condition where the force of blood against the blood vessel walls is too strong and can lead to various complications.

I

Impostor syndrome - A condition where individuals doubt their achievements.

Incision and Drainage - A minor procedure where a small cut is made to release pus or fluid from an infected area.

Incontinence pad - A pad worn to absorb urine or stool leaks, used by people with bladder or bowel control issues. It is also used to absorb any bodily fluid leakage during certain procedures.

Incubator - A machine that keeps newborn babies, especially premature ones, warm and protected while they grow stronger.

Infectious Peritonitis - Inflammation of the peritoneum (the lining of the abdominal cavity) due to infection, often presenting with severe abdominal pain and fever.

Inframammary - The area under the breast.

Internal Medicine - A branch of medicine that focuses on diagnosing and treating diseases in adults.

Intern - A new doctor in their first year of hospital work after medical school. It is a training position where they work under supervision.

Intravenous (IV) - Giving fluids or medicine directly into a vein, using a needle or small tube.

Intraosseous (IO) - A method of giving fluids or medicine directly into the bone, when veins are hard to access, usually in emergencies.

K

Kawasaki - A rare disease in children that causes fever, rash, and redness of the lips and tongue, as well as neck swelling, which can also have complications affecting the heart if not treated properly.

L

Labour room - A hospital room where a woman gives birth.

Laparoscopy - A type of surgery using small incisions and a camera-guided instrument.

Local anaesthetic - Medicine that numbs a small part of the body so a person doesn't feel pain during minor procedures.

Leukaemia - A group of cancers affecting the blood and bone marrow, marked by the uncontrolled production of abnormal white blood cells.

Lymphoma - A type of cancer that starts in the lymphatic system, which is part of the body's immune system.

M

Malignancy - Another word for cancer; a harmful mass or swelling, or uncontrolled division of cells that can spread to other parts of the body

Mastectomy - A surgical procedure to remove one or both breasts, usually to treat or prevent breast cancer.

Mediastinal Rhabdomyosarcoma - A rare cancer that starts in muscle tissue in the chest area (between the lungs), more common in children or teens.

Medical student syndrome - When medical students start thinking they have the diseases they're learning about, often due to stress or anxiety.

Meningitis - inflammation of the protective layers around the brain and spinal cord, often caused by infection. It can be serious or life-threatening.

Metabolic pathways - The chemical steps inside the body that turn food into energy and help in other bodily processes.

Metastases - Cancer cells that have spread from the original spot to other parts of the body, like the lungs, bones, or brain, for example.

Missed Miscarriage - When a baby dies in the womb, but the body hasn't shown signs like bleeding yet.

Murmur - An extra or unusual sound heard when listening to the heart. It can be harmless or a sign of a heart problem.

N

NICU(Neonatal Intensive Care Unit) - A special hospital unit that cares for very sick or premature newborn babies.

Necrotic - Dead tissue in the body, usually caused by poor blood supply, infection, or injury etc.

Neonatology - A branch of medicine that cares for newborn babies, especially those who are sick or born early.

Nephrologist - A doctor who specialises in treating kidney problems and diseases.

Nodule - A small lump or bump in the body. It can be harmless or may indicate a disease.

O

Obstetrics and Gynaecology (OBGYN) - The medical specialty that deals with pregnancy, childbirth, and the health of the female reproductive system.

Olfactory nerve - The nerve responsible for sense of smell. It sends smell signals from the nose to the brain.

On-call - A doctor who's on-call receives and responds to calls from the emergency or ward about patients they need to check and attend to for the duration that they're assigned. It may be eight, twelve, or even twenty-four hours at a stretch.

Oncology - The branch of medicine that focuses on the diagnosis and treatment of cancer.

Ophthalmology - The field of medicine that deals with eye health, vision problems, and eye surgery.

Orthopaedics - The branch of medicine that treats problems with bones, joints, muscles, and the spine.

OSCE - A practical exam for medical students to demonstrate their skills with patients, such as physical examination or communication skills.

P

Pain crisis - A sudden attack of pain, often seen in sickle cell disease, due to blocked blood flow to a particular organ or bone.

Palpation - A technique where a doctor uses their hands to feel the body to check for tenderness, lumps, or organ size for example.

Palliative care - Medical care focused on relieving pain and symptoms in serious illnesses, especially when a cure is not possible.

Panic disorder - A mental health condition where a person has repeated, unexpected panic attacks with symptoms like chest pain, sweating, and fear.

Paramedic - A highly trained emergency responder who gives medical care before the patient reaches the hospital.

Parastomal Hernia - A bulge or lump near a surgical opening (called a stoma), caused by tissue pushing through weak muscles. Common after certain bowel surgeries.

Paraesthesia - An abnormal skin sensation, such as tingling or numbness, including feeling like one is being poked by "pins and needles."

Paediatrics - The branch of medicine that deals with the health and medical care of babies, children, and teenagers.

Paediatric Oncology - The medical specialty focused on diagnosing and treating cancers in children and adolescents.

Pansystolic murmur - A heart sound heard during the entire squeezing phase of the heartbeat, often linked to valve problems.

Pelvic Inflammatory Disease (PID) - An infection of the female reproductive organs, usually caused by infection, leading to pain, fever, or infertility.

Pathologist - A medical doctor who diagnoses diseases by examining tissues, cells, and body fluids, often through laboratory tests and biopsies.

Pathology - The study of disease, including its causes, mechanisms, and effects on body tissues and organs.

Percussion - When a doctor taps on the body to listen for changes in sound that might indicate problems, such as fluid in the lungs, for example.

Pharmacology - The study of medicines and how they work in the body, including how they're absorbed, used, and eliminated.

Physical examination - When a doctor checks the body by looking, touching, listening, and sometimes tapping to find signs of illness.

Physiology - The branch of science that studies the normal functions of the body and how organs and systems work.

Pneumonia - An infection of the lungs causing cough, fever, chest pain, and difficulty breathing.

Postoperative period - The time after surgery.

Post-Traumatic Stress Disorder (PTSD) - A mental health condition that can develop after experiencing a terrifying or traumatic event, with symptoms like flashbacks, anxiety and nightmares.

Psychiatry - The branch of medicine that diagnoses and treats mental health disorders, such as depression, anxiety, or schizophrenia, among others.

Pulmonology - The branch of medicine that is related to diseases of the lungs and respiratory system.

Pulseless Electrical Activity (PEA) - A medical emergency where the heart has electrical activity on a monitor, but no actual pulse or pumping activity.

Q

Qur'an - The holy book of Islam, believed by Muslims to be the word of God as revealed to the Prophet Muhammad (peace be upon him).

R

Ramadan - A holy month in Islam where Muslims fast from sunrise to sunset, focusing on prayer, self-discipline, giving, and spiritual growth.

Resident - A doctor who has graduated from medical school and is now training in a specific specialty under supervision in the hospital.

Resuscitation - Medical interventions aimed at restoring vital functions, typically used in life-threatening emergencies.

Return of Spontaneous Circulation (ROSC) - When the heart starts beating effectively on its own again after it had stopped, often after CPR.

Rounds - When a group of doctors visit patients together, discussing treatment plans and checking progress.

S

Scalpel - A small, very sharp knife that surgeons use during operations.

Sedation - Medicine used to relax or make you sleepy during a procedure or other situations.

Sepsis - A life-threatening reaction to infection, where the body's response causes widespread inflammation and organ dysfunction.

Septic abortion - A serious infection that can occur after a miscarriage or unsafe abortion, requiring urgent treatment.

Seroma - A pocket of clear fluid that can collect under the skin usually after surgery.

Shift Captain - The senior doctor or leader responsible for managing a medical team during a specific shift in the hospital.

Shock - A life-threatening condition where the body doesn't get enough blood flow, leading to organ failure if not treated quickly.

Sickle cell anaemia - A genetic blood disorder where red blood cells are misshapen like sickles, causing pain, anaemia, and other complications.

Spinal Stenosis - Narrowing of the spaces within the spine, which can put pressure on nerves and cause pain or weakness.

Sports Medicine - A medical field focused on treating injuries and conditions related to physical activity and sports.

Stethoscope - A tool doctors use to listen to the heart, lungs, or belly.

Stroke - A medical emergency where blood flow to part of the brain is blocked by a clot or bleeding, causing brain damage.

SVT (Supraventricular Tachycardia) - A condition involving an abnormally fast heart rhythm originating above the heart's ventricles.

S4 - An extra sound heard when listening to the heart, it can mean the heart is stiff or overworked.

T

Thrill - A vibration you can feel with your hand when touching the skin over a blood vessel or heart. It usually means blood is flowing abnormally, often due to a heart or vessel problem.

Tonsillectomy - Surgery to remove the tonsils, often done for repeated sore throats, snoring, or breathing difficulties while sleeping.

Tuberculosis - A bacterial infection, most often affecting the lungs, caused by *Mycobacterium Tuberculosis.* It can affect other organs too.

U

Ultrasound - A test that uses sound waves to create images of the inside of the body. It is used during pregnancy to examine the baby's growth and in emergencies to check for any fluid from bleeding or injury, for example.

Underwater Seal - A type of chest drain that helps remove air or fluid from the chest and prevents it from re-entering.

Urinary Catheter - A thin tube put into the bladder to drain urine, mostly used when someone can't pee on their own.

Urinary Incontinence - The unintentional loss of bladder control, leading to leakage of urine.

V

Vascular surgery - Surgery on blood vessels, like arteries and veins, to fix problems such as blockages, aneurysms, or injuries etc.

Ventilator - A machine that helps someone breathe when they're too sick to breathe on their own.

Vital signs - Basic body measurements like heart rate, blood pressure, temperature, breathing rate, and oxygen saturation that indicate how the body is doing.

Vitally unstable - When a person's vital signs are very abnormal and the body is struggling to survive.

W

Ward - A hospital room or section where patients stay during treatment.

A TOKEN OF GRATITUDE TO

The Almighty, for the gift of dreams that inspire, knowledge that enlightens, and wisdom to share with others.

Professor Yousif Eltayeb, for believing in the potential of this project and offering constant support.

Mrs Sabeena Salam, whose spark lit the way for this endeavour, and whose guidance, supervision and steadfast leadership brought this work to life.

The remarkable team behind this project-

Dr Mariyam Thahira, who first envisioned and coordinated it;

Dr Suhaila Ahmed, Dr Maryam Rahmatullah, Dr Anaam Parveen and Dr Fathimah Aaliya Anwar, for their incredible ideas and enthusiasm throughout the process; by playing various roles including planning, compiling, editing, reviewing, forming glossary and much more.

Dr Faatimah Maryam Muzammil, Dr Manal Saleem, Dr Sarah Masood, Dr Raabeah Fatma Jafri, Dr Aisha Ismail Makandar, Dr Namra Fatma Jafri and Dr Shiza Ali, for editing and reviewing as well as creating the glossary with unwavering dedication and care.

Dr Saima Liyakat Khan, whose illustrations capture the heart of every theme with grace and precision.

The publishing team, for their meticulous edits, timely service, and professional touch.

The healthcare professionals, trainees, and students who shared their stories with such honesty, vulnerability, and insight.

The patients whose lives continue to teach us the finest lessons in both science and empathy.

And finally, to you, the reader. Thank you for spending time with these voices. May their words stay with you and inspire a deeper appreciation for the human spirit behind every white coat.

www.ingramcontent.com/pod-product-compliance
Lightning Source LLC
LaVergne TN
LVHW100306210926
848480LV00003B/1033